EVOCATIVE IMAGES

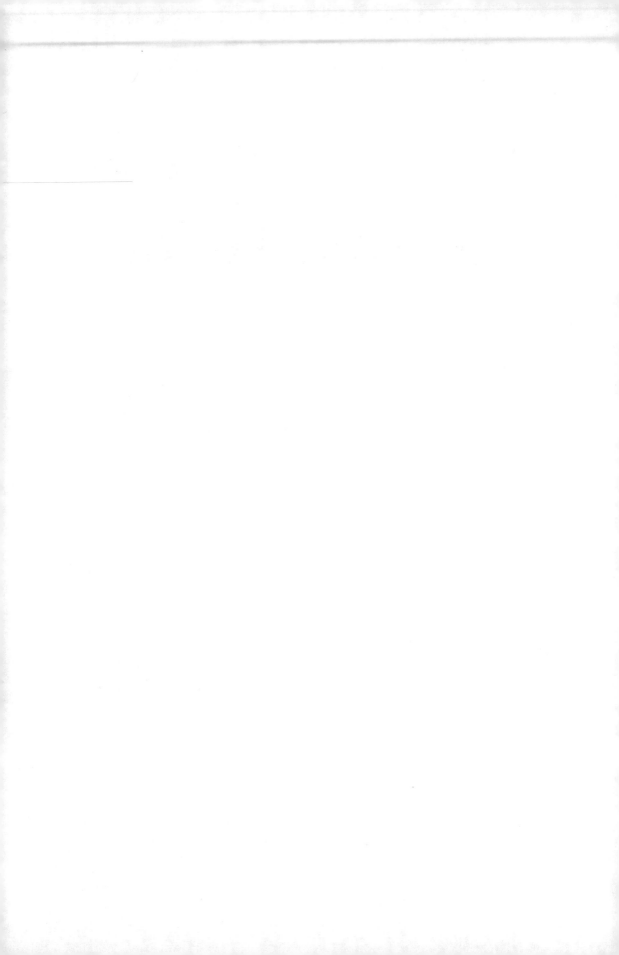

EVOCATIVE IMAGES

THE THEMATIC APPERCEPTION TEST AND THE ART OF PROJECTION

EDITED BY
LON GIESER AND MORRIS I. STEIN

AMERICAN PSYCHOLOGICAL ASSOCIATION
Washington, DC

Published by
American Psychological Association
750 First Street, NE
Washington, DC 20002

Copies may be ordered from
APA Order Department
P.O. Box 92984
Washington, DC 20090-2984

In the U.K., Europe, Africa, and the Middle East, copies may be ordered from
American Psychological Association
3 Henrietta Street
Covent Garden, London
WC2E 8LU England

Typeset in Century Schoolbook by EPS Group Inc., Easton, MD

Printer: Sheridan Press, Ann Arbor, MI
Dust jacket designer: DRI Consulting, Chevy Chase, MD
Technical/Production Editor: Amy J. Clarke

Library of Congress Cataloging-in-Publication Data
Evocative images : the thematic apperception test and the art of projection /
    edited by Lon Gieser and Morris I. Stein.—1st ed.
        p.   cm.
    Includes bibliographical references and index.
    ISBN 1-55798-579-0 (hardcover : acid-free paper)
    1. Thematic Apperception Test.   I. Gieser, Lon, 1955–   .
II. Stein, Morris Isaac, 1921–   .
    BF698.8.T5E96   1999
    155.2′844—dc21   99-25182
                                                                            CIP

British Library Cataloguing-in-Publication Data
A CIP record is available from the British Library.

Printed in the United States of America
First Edition

To Kate and Max.
L. G.

To Sara and David.
M. I. S.

Contents

Foreword:
Harry's Compass

Henry A. Murray—Harry to me—loved to explore. He started as a boy climbing Swiss mountains and played alone at the seashore, where he sailed his little ship off on mysterious voyages. His mature life, of course, was spent exploring personality at the Harvard Psychological Clinic at Harvard University. Whether in Switzerland, on imaginary high seas, or traveling through the mind, Harry always wanted a compass in hand. He was a careful and tidy explorer and liked to go from a well-supplied base camp out into the unknown, carrying tools to make maps and keep logs. The Thematic Apperception Test (TAT) became his steady companion throughout his life, his compass leading him along unexplored paths.

Gerald Holton demonstrated the process of scientific discovery, showing that outstanding scientists use visual, metaphorical, and thematic means at the beginning of their searches to clarify their ideas before rigorously testing them with up-to-date statistical and scientific methods.[1] The TAT certainly provided Harry with visual, metaphorical, and thematic details as he formulated his theories and decided on the arrangement of subsystems within his regnant system of personology.

Harry would be thrilled to find that his compass has proved useful to such a disparate group of exploring scientists as appear in this volume. He would be excited by the range and detail of their projects and be nodding his head in approval, smiling, and—I am sure—making mordant comments as he read how the TAT has been examined vis-à-vis such variegated subjects as art, literature, and science. There is his compass again, used in exploring clinical and research problems, social personality theory, cross-cultural psychology, and narrative therapy. How he would love to be back with his old colleagues at the Harvard Psychological Clinic! I can hear him bantering and laughing with Leopold Bellak, Robert Holt, David McClelland, Saul Rosenzweig, Ed Shneidman, Moe Stein, and Robert White, as they sit together in some distant imaginary intellectual space trying to read together the information coming from that ever-challenging instrument, the TAT.

Harry had already set a fine example in using the TAT in many different settings for many different purposes. Although he often followed leads that were unfruitful, he never discarded his TAT.

One compass search that led him to a dead end was made with a set called the TAT II. Harry designed the pictures of the TAT II to elicit Jungian archetypes. He had a tender feeling for the TAT II. He showed me

---

[1] See G. Holton (1996, Spring), "On the Art of Scientific Imagination," in *Daedalus, Journal of the Academy of Arts and Sciences: Managing Innovation,* pp. 183–208.

the pictures with pride when we were first married. Did archetypes, he had wondered, activate thinking in predictable directions?

The TAT II was a set of 20 complicated and supposedly ambiguous pictures. They were rich in detail and color and had inlays that were out of proportion to the main picture. Some were pastels, whereas others were brightly colored and set in foreign countries like Mexico. These cards demonstrated the presence of Jungian archetypes, no matter what the cultural setting. As always, Harry had a detailed, intricate, and probably impossible research scheme to test the theory that "the anima," "the old man," "puer," and so forth lived in and moved everyone.

Card 20 could hardly be called ambiguous, that is, if you knew Harry, Christiana Morgan, Carl Jung, and Toni Wolff's history. The central picture is of Harry and Christiana's tower on the Parker River (modeled after Jung's tower at Bollingen on Lake Geneva, Switzerland). In the upper right hand corner is an inlay of an old man, bearded and wearing a fedora. In the lower left hand corner is an inlay of a large, dark-haired, dark-eyed, two-faced woman. Both her profile and full face depict an anima if I ever saw one. In contrast, Card 3 is a pale watercolor of a couple of frogs sitting at the base of a waterfall, which never brought any archetype immediately to my mind. Harry once asked Holt to make a blind analysis of responses to the TAT II, but Holt (personal communication, May 22, 1996) reported, as he remembered it, that the cards did not seem to evoke Jungian images or themes. This particular theoretical search using the TAT II was abandoned, in part, for lack of promising results.

In a similar vein, Harry once invented a set of TAT cards based on stories in the New Testament. He wanted to see which characters participants identified with and the role of Christian symbols on spontaneous thought.

Not only did Harry use the TAT to explore major novel theories that would contribute to his understanding of personology, but he also used the TAT for specific practical tasks. For instance, he put together varying sets of TATs for use by the military in World War 2.

One set was designed for the U.S. Navy, with pictures of men in naval uniforms facing problems common to men on ships at sea. Harry examined their responses for clues to prospective behavior. Combat officers and U.S. Air Force pilots each had their own TAT. Of course, the U.S. Office of Strategic Services used the regularly published TAT extensively in choosing undercover men for the military, scoring responses for energy, speed, and control. Harry developed a Chinese TAT in Kunming, China, where he was sent by the Office of Strategic Services toward the end of the war to select paratroopers for the Chinese Army. He even designed an intriguing set of TAT cards to probe the psyches of Russians in wartime. I do not know who was supposed to take these tests, Russians or American spies going to Russia, but the models in the pictures were of Russian men in business suits and ties working in offices around tables. One card showed a man flying first class. (Harry, always forward looking, seemed to be anticipating present-day Russia.) Harry's daughter, Josephine, told me that he designed a set of TAT cards to draw out Ethiopians, but neither of us can remember why he was inspired to look at the psyches of Ethiopians.

From the beginning, Harry regarded an individual's responses to the TAT as a cognitive process, a test of imagination that is a conscious reasoning selection of emotional memories. In the last years of his life, spurred by our friendship and conversations with Larry Kohlberg and Howard Gardner, Harry began to concentrate on logical and moral development when interpreting TATs. Central aspects of psychoanalytic thought, such as defense mechanisms, became his secondary interest. Just as he had once tried to find Jungian archetypes, now he was using his compass to explore cognitive processes in TAT responses. How, he wondered, did emotions and logic work together in a story? He carefully analyzed the individual's selected objects within the chosen field and noted how they were perceived (and misperceived) and how schemas were built. Was the story just a string of "and then . . . and then . . . and then . . . ," or were complex moral issues interwoven into the storyline?

Harry would take TAT responses I brought home from my diagnostic testing of inner-city children and give them a quick interpretation, as he used to do at the Harvard Psychological Clinic, sorting out needs and press. He would then try and understand how the children used categories and how complex the relationships were among these categories. He always looked for animism in replies, but now he looked for animism as typical of a certain stage of cognitive development. He looked to see if the children's responses were in simple dichotomies. Or were the children describing a story with superordinate and complex groupings? How, he asked, did the children discriminate among classes of people? Were categories repeated with each card, or was there development and flexibility in playing with them? We were both so intrigued by this exploration that we began to write together a textbook on the relationship of thinking and feeling, but this project became so complex and demanding that Harry preferred finishing his biography of Herman Melville and I shifted to trying to deliver the message in a novel.

Finally, before his devastating strokes, Harry was concentrating on semiotics and linguistics, approaching the interpretation of the TAT with another and different theoretical stance: studying words and symbols, semantics and syntax, and their relations to emotional control. Harry paid particular attention to the length and complexity of each sentence.

Harry believed in using multiform procedures to test assumptions; but in the single procedure, the TAT, he found one test that continually provided him with a way to explore multiformed aspects of the developing mind. For Harry, there was no set way to use or interpret the TAT and, for that matter, no set TAT. How, I wonder now, would Harry be using the TAT to explore chaos theory?

CAROLINE C. MURRAY

Acknowledgments

We are grateful to innumerable individuals whose work on the Thematic Apperception Test (TAT) has inspired our own: first, to Henry A. Murray, whose psychological genius and vision gave birth to the animating idea for the TAT; next, to some of the TAT's other shapers, developers, and advocates: Murray's close collaborator, Christiana Morgan; Robert White, who was an invaluable consultant for this book; Nevitt Sanford; Sylvan Tompkins; Frederick Wyatt; David Rapaport; Merton Gill; Roy Schafer; William Henry; David Shakow; Ruth Markmann; Shirley Mitchell; Samuel Thal, and Jurgen Reusch. We also include here four authors of this volume: Saul Rosenzweig, Leopold Bellak, Robert Holt, and Edwin Shneidman. We are saddened by the recent death of another author, David McClelland, who, more than anyone else, extended the TAT approach in the social sciences.

We are deeply indebted to the many people who contributed to the publication of this book. Barbara Madsen, typist extraordinaire, prepared our manuscript. Donald Freedheim introduced us to APA Books. Gary VandenBos, APA Publisher, and Julia Frank-McNeil, Director of APA Books, gave our project their blessing. Our APA Books editors—colleagues, Margaret Schlegel (Acquisitions), Linda McCarter (Development), and Amy Clarke (Technical/Production), showed us how to do things the right way and shepherded the book through the press. Our fellow authors gave us their best, did not dodge too many deadlines, and agreed with our proposal to donate all royalties to the Henry A. Murray Research Center at Harvard University (Radcliffe College, 10 Garden Street, Cambridge, MA 02139).

We are very fortunate to have families and friends who provided us with their love and support and helped us to keep things in perspective.

To paraphrase Yogi Berra, we would like to thank everyone who made these acknowledgments necessary.

Contributors

David M. Abrams, PhD, Clinic Director, Community Counseling and Mediation, New York, and Department of Clinical Psychology, City University of New York and Yeshiva University, New Rochelle

James William Anderson, PhD, Division of Psychology, Department of Psychiatry and Behavioral Sciences, Northwestern University Medical School, Chicago, IL

Leopold Bellak, MD, Emeritus Professor of Psychiatry, Albert Einstein College of Medicine, Yeshiva University, New York, and Postdoctoral Program in Psychoanalysis and Psychotherapy, New York University, New York

Guiseppe Costantino, PhD, Sunset Park Mental Health Center, Lutheran Medical Center, Fordham University, and St. John's University, Brooklyn, NY

Richard H. Dana, PhD, Regional Research Institute for Human Services, Portland State University, Portland, OR

Lon Gieser, PhD, independent practice, Upper Montclair and Summit, NJ

Hubert J. M. Hermans, PhD, Department of Psychology, University of Nijmegen, the Netherlands

Robert R. Holt, PhD, Professor of Psychology Emeritus, New York University, Truro, MA

Robert G. Malgady, PhD, Program for Quantitative Studies, New York University, New York

David C. McClelland, PhD, deceased, formerly of Department of Psychology, Harvard University, Cambridge, MA

Wesley G. Morgan, PhD, Department of Psychology, University of Tennessee, Knoxville

Caroline C. Murray, EdD, Lecturer Emerita, Harvard University Medical School, Nantucket, MA

Saul Rosenzweig, PhD, Department of Psychology, Washington University, St. Louis, MO

Edwin S. Shneidman, PhD, Professor of Thanatology Emeritus, Neuropsychiatric Institute, University of California, Los Angeles

Morris I. Stein, PhD, Professor Emeritus of Psychology, New York University, New York

David G. Winter, PhD, Department of Psychology, University of Michigan, Ann Arbor

Part I

Introduction

1

An Overview of the Thematic Apperception Test

Lon Gieser and Morris I. Stein

In the early 1930s, Henry A. Murray, Director of the Harvard Psychological Clinic at Harvard University, became fascinated with the potential of storytelling for delving into the human psyche to better understand psychodynamics and behavior. Murray had trained as a surgeon, earned a PhD in biochemistry, immersed himself in the arts, and studied psychology independently. He interpreted the discoveries of Sigmund Freud and his own mentor Carl Jung as supporting the conviction that "in the human being imagination is more fundamental than perception" (Murray, 1951/1953, p. 6). Consequently, Murray devoted himself to furthering their investigation of "dreams, fantasies, creative production—and projection—all of which are primarily emotional and dramatic, such stuff as myths are made of" (p. 7). After much experimentation with evocative images, Murray, along with Christiana Morgan and other clinic staff, fashioned the now classic Thematic Apperception Test (TAT).

The TAT consists of 30 cards, each showing an ambiguous black and white picture of a situation or event. Individuals are asked to make up stories for the pictures. There is also a blank card for which individuals are asked to create their own scene, about which they are then asked to tell a story. Designated sets of 20 pictures are administered to men and women; two other sets are administered to boys and girls. Murray recommended that the TAT be administered in two 1-hour sessions, consisting of 10 cards each. Today, clinical psychologists typically use 10 cards or less during a single session. Story themes can reveal information about one's relationships with lovers, friends, parents, and authority figures. Insight can be gained regarding an individual's life view, including self-concept and characteristic coping styles in facing emotional conflict.

Background

The TAT was introduced beyond the Harvard Psychological Clinic in an article by C. Morgan and Murray (1935/1981); they wrote that the TAT is

> based on the well recognized fact that when someone attempts to interpret a complex social situation he is apt to tell as much about himself

3

as he is about the phenomenon on which his attention is focused. At such times, the person is off his guard, since he believes he is merely explaining objective occurrences. To one with 'double hearing,' however, he is exposing certain inner forces and arrangements, wishes, fears, and traces of past experiences." (p. 390)

C. Morgan and Murray "anticipated that in the performance of the storytelling task a subject would necessarily be forced to project some of his own fantasies into the material and so reveal his more pressing underlying needs" (p. 391).

TAT stories were analyzed by C. Morgan and Murray according to Murray's conceptualization of personality. The storyteller is assumed to most identify with one character in a picture. This character becomes a story's protagonist (*hero*). Forces or motivational drives emanating from within the hero are termed *needs*. Environmental forces or situations affecting the expression of needs are called *press*. The interaction of needs and press results in an emotional *outcome*. Behavior resulting from the interaction of needs, press, and outcome is termed *thema*. Discovering patterns of themas in a series of stories provides insight into the core of the storyteller's personality.

Two illustrative case studies are provided. C. Morgan and Murray (1935/1981) concluded that the TAT is useful for "understanding of the deeper levels of a personality" (p. 401) and therefore could be helpful in expediting the process of psychoanalysis for patients, particularly young adults who did not need or could not afford a long course of therapy.

Development, Scoring, and Controversies

The TAT's development occurred as part of Murray's monumental study *Explorations in Personality* (Murray, 1938). Fifty Harvard undergraduates were assessed by the staff of the Harvard Psychological Clinic. The project was groundbreaking, first, in turning clinical psychology's focus to signs of strength and competence in personality as well as to symptoms and pathology. Second, an innovative "multiform" method was advanced. An assessment battery comprising a variety of interviews, questionnaires, and several new tests of imagination and abilities was used for each participant. In addition, a "diagnostic council" of researchers collaborated in combining the findings to form an in-depth profile for each participant. Third, *Explorations* presents Murray's theory of *personology*: This sophisticated conceptualization of psychodynamics is aimed at capturing the complexity and uniqueness of each individual's personality. It includes the systematic delineation of 29 needs, of 20 presses, and their possible interaction. *Explorations* demonstrates the TAT's value in the extensive case study approach advocated by personology. The use of the TAT in this context is exemplified by Robert White's (1975, 1981) work, beginning with his contribution to *Explorations* (White, 1938).

Murray found existing paper-and-pencil tests of personality insufficient and too simple to provide the desired understanding of the whole person. One projective test, the Rorschach, was already in use and rapidly growing in popularity. It contains several basic desiderata. It was based on perception—an area of human behavior that is usually studied in the laboratory. The test is scored for specific variables that could be quantified and assembled into profiles, which could then be interpreted to yield a meaningful picture of a person's psychodynamics. Such information could also be used in planning and facilitating the course of the individual's psychotherapy.

The TAT had all that the Rorschach had and more. Whereas the clinician used Rorschach data to infer personality dynamics from perception, the TAT could be used to infer personality dynamics from apperception. The Rorschach inferred psychodynamics from how the person saw the world (see the manifest in Rorschach cards); the TAT inferred psychodynamics from how the person understood and made meaningful people's motives, intentions, and expectations, in social situations. All of this was accomplished through a time-honored technique that people have used over many generations in their attempts to understand themselves and their fellow human beings, namely, the story. Add the "projective hypothesis" (Frank, 1939) to storytelling and for a good number of people, the TAT enjoyed immediate face validity.

The TAT and Rorschach both had scoring systems. For the Rorschach, it was essentially a series of shorthand symbols that reflected what was involved in the individual's perceptions. The TAT need–press scoring system, however, was rather complicated and elaborate. Just as with the Rorschach, the variables could be quantified. But whereas the Rorschach variables were central to the test, TAT variables were not that critical to garner information from the stories told for the pictures. One could use one's own theoretical system of personality dynamics.

Both the Rorschach and the TAT suffered from the same Achilles heel—both were described as tests; as such, they had to adhere to and fulfill the standards for psychological tests, specifically, reliability and validity. Case studies and anecdotes of how the TAT and the Rorschach were important to the understanding of the individual, even though they did not fulfill statistical desiderata, did not convince the whole psychological audience but appealed to a good number.

Explorations in Personality could be accepted by diverse groups of psychologists who might disagree with each other on various theoretical issues. But when it came to the TAT, it seemed that the audience boiled down to just two irreconcilable groups. One group, psychometrically oriented, identified strongly with the use of statistics to check on the test's reliability and validity. They argued strongly and consistently that tests like the TAT did not meet psychometric standards and therefore did not deserve to be called tests; they should not be used diagnostically or for research purposes (Eysenck, 1968).

In the second group, consisting of those who were more accepting of the TAT, were mostly clinicians who chose to ignore or disagree with the

psychometrists. Some in this group argued that tests meeting psychometricians' standards fractionate the person into meaningless units that do
not do justice to the uniqueness of the whole person. They also believed
that even standardized tests do not avoid the problems of the social de-
sirability of responses. Also some clinicians liked the idea that the TAT
was not a test because a test implies "evaluation"—always interfering
with the possibility of establishing rapport with the patient. In such a
clinician's hands, the TAT is a stimulus, a method of eliciting and gathering information in a nonthreatening manner. It therefore facilitates communication between psychologist and patient. With such experiences in
mind, the TAT might have been better titled the "thematic apperception
educator" (*eductor* is the word preferred by Murray [1967][1] or the "thematic apperception technique.")

The TAT was first distributed by the Harvard Psychological Clinic in
1936. It was revised three more times before the set of cards and manual
used today were published in 1943. By this time, Murray (1943) claimed
that

> the TAT is a method of revealing to the interpreter some of the domi-
> nant drives, emotions, sentiments, complexes and conflicts of person-
> ality. Special value resides in its power to expose underlying inhibited
> tendencies which a subject or patient is not willing to admit or cannot
> admit because he is unconscious of them. (p. 3)

The TAT participant was portrayed as unknowingly producing an "X-ray
picture of his inner self" (p. 4).

The manual recommends the quantitative need–press scoring scheme.
In addition to commenting on the TAT's utility in personality research and
clinical diagnosis, Murray (1943) again noted that "the technique is especially recommended as a preface to a series of psychotherapeutic interviews or to a shorter psychoanalysis" (p. 3).

The TAT quickly gained popularity in clinical practice. Since 1946,
using surveys, psychologists have consistently found that the TAT is used
by a majority of clinical psychologists; the clinicians ranked it among the
top four or five tests in most settings (Archer, Maruish, Imhof, & Piotrowski, 1991; Haynes & Peltier, 1985; Lubin, Wallis, & Praine, 1971; Piotrowski & Keller, 1989; Piotrowski, Sherry, & Keller, 1985; Piotrowski &
Zalewski, 1993; Sundberg, 1961; Watkins, Campbell, Nieberding, & Hallmark, 1995). It usually is preceded by the Wechsler Adult Intelligence
Scale (WAIS), the Minnesota Multiphasic Personality Inventory (MMPI),
the Bender Gestalt Visual Motor Test, and the Rorschach Inkblot Test.

Most psychologists receive graduate training to use the TAT, although
there are uneven training standards between programs (Rossini & Moretti, 1997). Despite some decreased interest in projective techniques rel-

---

[1]Murray (1967) explained that methods like the TAT might be better named "eductors"
than projective tests; they are designed to "educe (draw forth) words, sentences or stories
as ground for verifiable or plausible inferences in regard to influential components of the
personality which the subject is either unable or unwilling to report" (p. 304).

ative to the development of objective tests (e.g., the Millon Clinical Multiaxial Inventory and tests for assessing neuropsychological impairment), the TAT, along with the MMPI and Rorschach, continues to be a reigning member of psychology's personality assessment triumvirate (Butcher & Rouse, 1996; Watkins et al., 1995).

Personality and social psychology researchers have thrived on the TAT, publishing several thousand articles (by 1950 over 100 articles and by 1971 over 1,800 articles; Groth-Marnat, 1997). The TAT has proven itself to be remarkably versatile. Given its capacity to evaluate several dimensions of personality, it is characterized as offering a "wide-band" approach (Rabin, 1968). Among areas of study, to list a few, are abnormal personality, delinquency, social attitudes, cognitive style, imaginative processes, family dynamics, emotional reactivity, sexual adjustment, achievement motivation, intimacy, aggression, creativity, level of affect, problem-solving skill, substance abuse, recovery from physical illness, and verbal fluency.

The TAT and TAT-type approaches are the most frequently used assessment devices for cross-cultural research (Retief, 1987). They have been used in military and industrial personnel selection (including use by the National Aeronautical and Space Administration and the Peace Corps), neuropsychological assessment, and forensic evaluation. The TAT has been used worldwide.

Our examination of the TAT's own story is further enlivened by the controversy its success has created. Despite its extensive use by psychologists, the TAT still does not have a consensual scoring system and set of norms. It still cannot meet the same standards of reliability and validity that objective tests such as the WAIS-R and MMPI-2 can. Efforts to make it do so, for the most part, have left it mired in a "psychometrician's quicksand" (Rossini & Moretti, 1997). The TAT's status as a test continues to be greatly debated.

The TAT's ambiguous nature invites psychologists to project their own approaches onto its purpose or use. For better or worse, it lends itself to intuitive interpretation based on subjective clinical experience. Robert White (personal communication, October 1996) reminisced about the early days of the TAT at the Harvard Psychological Clinic:

> Harry [Murray's] enthusiastic interpretation of the TAT was the climax, the Grand Finale, of each case presentation meeting at the Clinic. Harry could astonish us by giving an interpretation of the subject's TAT that was always brilliant—and sometimes may even have been right.

The TAT also welcomes quantitative scoring based on the varieties of competing methodologies and theoretical orientations now ranging from orthodox psychoanalysis to cognitive–behaviorism. As far back as 1950, there are several books based on psychodynamic theory offering alternate approaches to quantitative scoring. In a review of the TAT, Murstein (1963) was moved to remark that "there would seem to be as many thematic scoring systems as there are hairs in the beard of Rasputin" (p. 23).

Interrater reliability can be mitigated by clinicians taking different approaches to the TAT material. Because of the richness and complexity of the material, each clinician may tap into different but still potentially valid aspects of the same person. Although different reports may then have different areas of focus, all may possibly still have a high degree of clinical relevance (Groth-Marnat, 1997).

Some believe that the TAT is properly or best used along with other techniques in an assessment battery. Others prefer to evaluate its performance as an independent measure of motives. In addition, there is a dwindling minority who view it as a psychotherapeutic tool rather than as a test or scientific research instrument.

The TAT imagery—some of which is obviously of 1930s–1940s vintage—may be considered archetypal; the TAT is thus perceived as a timeless old standby. The very same pictures may strike someone else as antiquated and in desperate need of revision or replacement. Some would prefer more energized color pictures, whereas others believe the gloomy black and white tones are most effective. There are differing degrees of desire to modify the cards for cross-cultural use or select segments of the population, such as adolescents, older people, business executives, and so on. Nevertheless, no single alternative version, with the exception of Bellak's Children's Apperception Test, has yet gained acceptance nearly as wide as that of the TAT.

About This Book

In this book, we trace the history of the TAT from its conception to the present. We document the versatility of the TAT and derivative approaches in research, diagnosis, and psychotherapy. Prospects for future use and development are considered.

The historical foundations of the TAT are examined in chapters 2, 3, and 4. Chapter 2 conveys the spirit of the times in which the TAT was developed. The TAT's psychometric lineage is critically examined beyond previous cursory histories of its development. One of the authors, Morris Stein, was Murray's graduate assistant at the Harvard Psychological Clinic in the early 1940s. In chapter 3, James Anderson tells how he first interviewed Murray about the TAT in 1973 and discussed it with him several times over the next 15 years of their friendship until Murray's death in 1988. Biographical information about Murray, including discussion of his extramarital affair with C. Morgan, is also provided. Controversy regarding C. Morgan's role in the origin of the TAT and the removal of her name from authorship of the test is addressed. Anderson's interviews are especially significant in light of Murray's ambivalent relationship with the TAT. Murray did not want to be identified with the common perfunctory mechanical use of the TAT to make reductionistic interpretations. For this reason, Murray did not choose to focus on the TAT in interviews with Forrest Robinson (personal communication, April 4, 1995) for his authorized biography. There is no other direct account of Murray's experiences with the development of the TAT.

In chapter 4, Saul Rosenzweig, who studied with Murray and C. Morgan, offers his perspective on the early clinical use of the TAT. He then focuses on his own work of compiling norms, systematizing TAT analysis, and applying the TAT to therapy and his studies of hypnotizability and creativity. For Murray (1943), "psychology was an expansive domain which spreads across the boundary between science and the arts" (p. 140). Chapter 5 explains the link between literary imagination and the storytelling approach to the TAT. One of the chapter's authors, Lon Gieser, interviewed Nevitt Sanford, a colleague of Murray's, who helped develop the TAT. Sanford points to the probable influence of the novelist Thomas Wolfe, which is corroborated by facts presented in the chapter. In chapter 6, Wesley Morgan describes each of the TAT pictures in use today and examines their artistic heritage. The processes involved in selecting and preparing the stimulus materials are elucidated. The artistic background of the stimulus materials is intended to aid contemporary interpretation of the stories told in response to them.

Part III explains what the TAT can measure and the TAT's role in research and clinical applications. In chapter 7, Edwin Schneidman, a later colleague of Murray's, presents the remarkable findings of a project in which 17 TAT experts were asked to independently interpret the same TAT protocol for a patient whom they had never met. The triumph of the TAT in psychodynamically skilled hands and the wealth of information it is capable of eliciting are well documented.

In chapter 8, Robert Holt, who worked with Murray at the Harvard Psychological Clinic in the 1940s, focuses on issues of reliability and validity in psychodiagnosis. He establishes the TAT's place in a diagnostic formulation in which ego psychology is central and a scientific multiform method is used. In chapter 9, David Winter describes the adaptation of the TAT into a group-administered research instrument for measuring individual personality variables, scored according to objectively defined criteria. He discusses the achievements of this approach from its origin by David McClelland in the late 1940s to its role in contemporary personality and social psychology.

In chapter 10, Morris Stein advances Murray's personological clinical approach in using the TAT. He describes a method of TAT interpretation in which the psychologist is not evaluative but aims at understanding the person who told the stories. In chapter 11, Leopold Bellak, who worked on TAT scoring with Murray at Harvard and developed his own widely used scoring system, explains the theory and practice of multidimensional diagnostic assessment with the TAT. Bellak champions integrating the TAT with psychotherapy, as was first proposed by C. Morgan and Murray. He discusses ways of doing so in crisis intervention and other forms of treatment. Bellak's colleague, David Abrams, concludes this section with chapter 12 and explains how the Bellak scoring system contributes to the clinical utility of the TAT. Abrams reviews the entire field of clinical–personality TAT research, ending with the TAT's current status.

The final section points to promising new directions for the application of thematic apperception techniques, including TATs other than Murray's. In chapter 13, the late David McClelland, who developed his own version of the TAT, sums up his life's work in extending the TAT approach in the study of human motivation, identifying themes in the life story, discovering cross-cultural themes, and evaluating vocational competencies. McClelland describes how unconscious motives, as determined by his "pure" TAT measure, influence important kinds of social behavior. He also reports how recent physiological research has begun to illustrate how these motives interact with hormonal processes. The unique capacity of the TAT approach to help psychologists continue to gain further understanding into human nature is elucidated.

Because the TAT and derived techniques have been so widely used for cross-cultural and multicultural populations, two chapters are devoted to this area. In chapter 14, Richard Dana describes the desired qualities for cross-cultural picture-story tests. Examples of cutting-edge work by Dana and others are given. Dana proposes a model for training, research, and practice to make the TAT method at least comparable with the Rorschach for multicultural populations. In chapter 15, Giuseppe Costantino and Robert Malgady present the Tell-Me-A-Story Test (TEMAS), an offspring of the TAT, developed for Hispanic children and adolescents and then expanded to include Blacks, Whites, and Asians. The TEMAS depicts ethnically pluralistic characters in familiar settings to make it relevant to American minorities as well as nonminorities. The psychometrics and clinical success of this test are shown.

Hubert Hermans (chap. 16) discusses the commonality of the storytelling approach of the TAT and narrative therapy. He provides a "polyphonic" perspective for TAT interpretation to better understand the multivoiced nature of the individual's self. A model for integrating the TAT with Hermans's narrative therapy approach is proposed.

We conclude this book with chapter 17 on the future of the TAT. Developments in theory, research, and practice are evaluated. Particular emphasis is placed on a burgeoning new field, the narrative study of human lives. Prospects for the TAT's use and metamorphosis are discussed. Our optimism regarding the continued adaptability of the TAT prevails.

Like Harry Murray, we view the TAT as an invaluable "compass" for explorations of personality that is best used following this motto: "Let not him who seeks cease until he finds, and when he finds he shall be astonished" (Murray, 1938, frontispiece).

References

Archer, R. P., Maruish, M., Imhof, E. A., & Piotrowski, C. (1991). Psychological test usage with adolescent clients: 1990 survey findings. *Professional Psychology: Research and Practice, 22*, 247–252.

Butcher, J. N., & Rouse, S. V. (1996). Personality: Individual differences and clinical assessment. *Annual Review of Psychology, 47*, 87–111.

Eysenck, H. J. (1968). *The scientific study of personality.* London: Routledge & K. Paul.

Frank, L. K. (1939). Projective methods for the study of personality. *Journal of Psychology,* *8,* 343–389.

Groth-Marnat, G. G. (1997). *Handbook of personality assessment* (3rd ed.). New York: Wiley.

Haynes, J. P., & Peltier, J. (1985). Patterns of practice with the TAT in juvenile forensic settings. *Journal of Personality Assessment, 3,* 26–29.

Lubin, B., Wallis, R., & Praine, C. (1971). Patterns of psychological test use in the United States: 1935–1969. *Professional Psychology: Research and Practice, 2,* 70–74.

Morgan, C. D., & Murray, H. A. (1981). A method for investigation of fantasies: The Thematic Apperception Test. In E. S. Shneidman (Ed.), *Endeavors in psychology: Selections from the personology of Henry A. Murray* (pp. 390–401). New York: Harper & Row. (Original work published 1935)

Murray, H. A. (Ed.). (1938). *Explorations in personality: A clinical and experimental study of fifty men of college age.* New York: Oxford University Press.

Murray, H. A. (1943). *Thematic Apperception Test: Manual.* Cambridge, MA: Harvard University Press.

Murray, H. A. (1953). In nomine diaboli. In J. Hillway & L. S. Mansfield (Eds.), *Moby Dick centennial essays* (pp. 3–23). Dallas, TX: Southern Methodist University Press. (Original work published 1951)

Murray, H. A. (1967). The case of Murr. In E. G. Boring & G. Lindzey (Eds.), *A history of psychology in autobiography* (pp. 283–310). New York: Appleton-Century-Crofts.

Murstein, B. I. (1963). *Theory and research in projective techniques (emphasizing the TAT).* New York: Wiley.

Piotrowski, C., & Keller, J. W. (1989). Psychological testing in outpatient mental health facilities: A national study. *Professional Psychology: Research and Practice, 20,* 423–425.

Piotrowski, C., Sherry, D., & Keller, J. W. (1985). Psychodiagnostic test usage: A survey of the Society for Personality Assessment. *Journal of Personality Assessment, 49,* 115–119.

Piotrowski, C., & Zalewski, C. (1993). Training in psychodiagnostic testing in APA-approved PsyD and PhD clinical training programs. *Journal of Personality Assessment, 61,* 394–405.

Rabin, A. I. (1968). *Projective techniques in personality assessment: A modern introduction.* New York: Springer.

Retief, A. (1987). Thematic apperception testing across cultures: Tests of selection versus tests of inclusion. *South African Journal of Psychology, 17,* 47–55.

Rossini, E. D., & Moretti, R. J. (1997). Thematic Apperception Test (TAT) interpretations: Practice recommendations from a survey of clinical psychology doctoral programs accredited by the American Psychological Association. *Professional Psychology: Research and Practice, 28,* 393–398.

Sundberg, N. (1961). The practice of psychological testing in clinical services in the United States. *American Psychologist, 16,* 79–83.

Watkins, C. E., Campbell, V. L., Nieberding, R., & Hallmark, R. (1995). Contemporary practice of psychological assessment by clinical psychologists. *Professional Psychology: Research and Practice, 26,* 54–60.

White, R. W. (1938). The case of Earnst. In H. A. Murray (Ed.), *Explorations in personality* (pp. 615–702). New York: Oxford University Press.

White, R. W. (1975). *Lives in progress: A study of the natural growth of personality* (3rd ed.). New York: Holt, Rinehart, & Winston.

White, R. W. (1981). Exploring personality the long way: The study of lives. In A. I. Rubin, J. Aranoff, A. M. Barclay, & R. A. Rucker (Eds.), *Further explorations in personality* (pp. 3–26). New York: Wiley.

Part II

Historical Foundations

2

The Zeitgeists and Events Surrounding the Birth of the Thematic Apperception Test

Morris I. Stein and Lon Gieser

What if Henry Murray had not existed, would there have been a Thematic Apperception Test (TAT)? This kind of "what if" question is grist for the mill for anyone interested in creativity. For those who believe that "man makes history," there would not have been a TAT without Murray. Those who believe that "history makes the man" would argue that just as James Watt was not critical to the development of the steam engine, if Murray had not lived, the TAT would have been developed by someone else. Those who knew Murray and were acquainted with his genius do not believe the second hypothesis one bit. Nevertheless, it is a hypothesis that must be entertained.

A Series of Transactions

The orientation here is that both theses—man makes history and history makes the man—are too simplistic. A more appropriate orientation is that creativity occurs in a social context; there are several players in this process. There is the "man" of man makes history, and there are others who serve as *intermediaries*—intimates, facilitators, mentors, advisers, critics (positive and negative), all of whom help move the course of events forward. There is also the audience to whom the communication or product is directed. As Walt Whitman (in Bartlett, 1980) said, "to have great poets, there must be great audiences too" (p. 577). Finally, there is the *zeitgeist,* those factors that constitute the "spirit of the times," which frequently exercise profound influences on shaping new developments and effecting their acceptance and survival.

As our thesis, the TAT is an outgrowth of a series of transactions between diverse people and events. In line with the spirit of this book, it behooves us to examine some of these events, so that readers can better appreciate the development of the TAT.

Murray's Start

Our story starts with Morton Prince. He initiated a chain of events that had important repercussions for Murray and the future of personality theory and research in the United States. Along about 1880, Prince took his mother, "who suffered from an undiagnosed neurotic disorder" (Triplet, 1992, p. 227), to Paris, France, for a consultation with Jean Charcot, pathologist and founder of neurology, at Salpêtrière. Prince remained so impressed with the use of a clinic for consultations and case demonstrations to help practitioners that more than 40 years later, he approached President A. Lawrence Lowell of Harvard University with the proposition to endow a similar clinic. Prince "was convinced that the research in psychopathology would flourish in a university setting, a comfortable remove from the distracting practical demands upon students at medical schools, the traditional locus of study in the field" (Robinson, 1992, p. 140). Lowell accepted the clinic endowment and appointed Prince for 1 year as a professor of abnormal psychology in the Department of Philosophy and Psychology.

With the planned establishment of a clinic, Prince needed a research assistant. Among the people he consulted was L. J. Henderson, a noted Harvard chemist who became crucial as an intermediary. Henderson recommended a young man—Henry A. Murray—who had done postgraduate research with him in biochemistry. Without further ado, Murray, at the age of 33 (Murray, 1967, p. 287), was appointed research associate in the Department of Philosophy and Psychology in 1926—the same year in which the Harvard Psychological Clinic was founded. By 1928, he was promoted to a nontenured professorship.

What is interesting about Murray's first appointment as a research associate (in the light of contemporary appointment procedures in academia) is that a search committee was not involved. Murray's educational credentials were not carefully reviewed, and the faculty did not realize that a candidate with a PhD in biochemistry had been selected for the position of Director of the Harvard Psychological Clinic. In fact, Murray himself "was the first to admit that he was unqualified for the job; though he had done a good deal of reading" (Robinson, 1992, p. 142) in psychology.[1]

Two years after Murray's appointment, Prince's health began to fail, so he retired in 1928. Who would his replacement be? Prince felt that Murray was the best person to succeed him. By this time, however, the faculty had learned the truth about Murray's educational credentials and questioned them. Some also objected to his interest in psychoanalysis. Edwin G. Boring, in particular, had hoped that Murray would be a more rigorous scientist and wanted someone more to his liking as the director of the clinic. Lowell, however, threw his support behind Murray; so Murray

---

[1]As one studies creative developments over the course of time, there is no hard and fast rule that creativity outcomes result when individuals and fields are matched precisely. As a prime example in this regard, whereas many engineers failed in their attempts to develop a workable telephone, Alexander Graham Bell, a teacher of the deaf who knew the workings of the inner ear, succeeded.

was appointed the clinic's director, starting with the academic year 1928–1929.

Despite tenuous support and even open hostility, Murray assumed his academic responsibilities with characteristic dedication and enthusiasm. A very popular teacher, he attracted many undergraduates to his courses, only to arouse further the suspicions of his detractors—How could a popular teacher be a good professor?

If the support for Murray in Harvard's Department of Psychology and Philosophy was flimsy,[2] he was almost completely isolated when it came to the broader scheme of things in American psychology. Robinson (1992) described the zeitgeist as follows:

> The American academy in the 1920s made no room for abnormal psychology and psychotherapy, which were condescended to as "applied" fields and relegated to the medical schools. Personality research was rarely undertaken on a systematic basis. The American Psychological Association had about a thousand members in 1928 (as compared with about 100,000 in 1990), most of them experimental in orientation. This is to say that they consciously emulated the methods and objectives of physical science. Cornell's Edward Titchener, reductionist par excellence and advocate of psychology as pure science, and John B. Watson, father of behaviorism, were dominant figures. Gestalt psychology had not yet taken root in this country. Freud and his followers were not unknown, but they had virtually no influence with leading academicians, who viewed them with suspicion. (p. 148)

Picture-Story Research

Given this state of affairs, it is not surprising that projective methods like the TAT had yet to find a foothold. There were, however, a few reports of picture-story research prior to the TAT. Tomkins (1947) cited four relatively unknown precursors, three of which involved participants creating stories for pictures (Brittain, 1907; Libby, 1908; Schwartz, 1932). The fourth was Clark's (1926) "phantasy" method for the psychoanalysis of narcissists, which relied solely on the patient's imagination.

Brittain (1907), in his study of imagination, presented a series of pictures to adolescent boys and girls and instructed them to write stories for the pictures. Brittain's findings focused on sex differences with regard to expressed interest, affective expression, and unity of plot. Brittain commented on how societal limits on social and physical activities for girls seemed to adversely affect their emotional life and imagination. His interpretation of the data did not address implications of the stories with regard to individual personality dynamics.

Libby (1908) investigated the imagination of children ages 10–14 compared with that of senior high school students. The children wrote stories for pictures. Libby observed that the stories of the older students were

---

[2]Murray did not receive tenure and full professorship until 1948.

more subjective than those of the younger ones, which he attributed primarily to further physiological development of the heart and brain.

Clark (1926) reported on the phantasy method for the psychoanalysis of narcissistic patients otherwise inaccessible to the analyst. He requested of such patients to imagine themselves as infants and to tell him the feelings, attitudes, and behaviors they believed young infants might have. Clark claimed that this emotional material evoked facilitated transference and thereby led to successful analyses.

Schwartz (1932), a psychiatrist, developed the Social Situation Picture Test as a means by which to expedite initial clinical interviews of juvenile delinquents. The test consists of eight pictures depicting scenes of a "moral nature"; these were presented to delinquent boys ages 10–12. One picture, for example, shows a boy fishing near a "no fishing" sign, whereas other boys in the background are apparently on their way to school. Schwartz asked a male juvenile delinquent to describe what he saw and what the boy in the picture was thinking. If the boy gave a simple objective account, Schwartz would conduct an inquiry as to the motives, thoughts, and probable actions of the main character, directly asking the boy what he would do if he were the boy in the picture. Schwartz's purpose was to get the boy to project aspects of his personality in his replies.

Thematic Apperception Test Beginnings

Murray was inconsistent with regard to giving credit for the TAT, sometimes citing influences in TAT publications, sometimes not (see Gieser & Morgan, chap. 5; and Morgan, chap. 6, this volume). None of the studies covered by Tomkins were ever cited by Murray himself. He may or may not have been acquainted with these antecedent storytelling techniques for the study of imagination or elicitation of fantasies. It is therefore difficult to place the TAT in a direct lineage. Nevertheless, Tomkins's history can be taken to imply that Schwartz's work served as a primary impetus for Murray to devise the TAT. Murstein (1963) went so far as to credit Schwartz with "creating the Thematic method of studying personality as we know it today" (p. 19).

Murray must have eventually become familiar with Schwartz's work (perhaps through Tomkins), but it should be emphasized that Murray began experimenting with apperceptive projective techniques beginning around 1930, well before Schwartz's article (see Anderson, chap. 3; and Gieser & Morgan, chap. 5, this volume). Whereas Schwartz's thematic method was a valuable contribution to psychology, his specialized test lacks three of the most significant qualities of the TAT: Its aim is to tap "root fantasies" of personality; its focus is on evoking emotion; and its element of ambiguity is designed to best produce projective processes.

Murray submitted the TAT's inaugural paper to Ernest Jones, editor of the *International Journal of Psychoanalysis* in 1934. Jones (personal communication, November 9, 1934) did not accept the paper for publication. He suggested that it was more suitable for a psychology journal because "[it] has a great deal to tell psychologists that is new to them, which is obviously its purpose rather than doing the same for analysts." Jones praised the TAT as an important link in the chain that must one day bind analysis and academic psychology, but he chided Murray for failing to acknowledge the earlier European projective techniques of Sandor Ferenczi (forced phantasies), Melanie Klein (play technique), and Hermann Rorschach (psychodiagnosis) as well as Jung's use of the picture method for eliciting material. Nevertheless, the only other projective test mentioned in the publication (Morgan & Murray, 1935) was the Rorschach.

According to Caroline C. Murray (personal communication, September 22, 1997), Harry Murray spoke to her of his interest in Carl Jung's (1904–1919/1973) studies in word association, which he began in the early 1920s. The experimental method of testing that Jung elaborated in these studies was used to reveal effectively significant groups of ideas in the unconscious, for which Jung coined the term *complexes*. Murray reviewed this work by Jung as having been a significant influence on the development of his own systematic methodological apperceptive studies. Later on, Morgan's artistic "visionary" experience with Jung influenced Murray's scientific work (see Anderson, chap. 3, this volume).

The article formally launching the TAT appeared in 1935 (Morgan & Murray, 1935). The findings in this article were part of the results of the first full-scale personological project completed by Murray and the staff of the Harvard Psychological Clinic, which was reported in *Explorations in Personality: A Clinical and Experimental Study of Fifty Men of College Age* (Murray, 1938). Murray and his research staff conducted the study with such intensity and extensity that the Harvard Psychological Clinic, then in the little house at 64 Plympton Street, was described as "wisteria on the outside and hysteria on the inside" (Robinson, 1992, p. 151).

Explorations is a monumental work that is a cornerstone of contemporary psychology. Before *Explorations*, dynamic psychology in the United States drew its inspiration and support from abroad or from emigrés— most notably Freud, Jung, Adler, Rank, Lewin, and Goldstein. In *Explorations*, Murray, with the help of his coworkers, selected the best of existing theories and knowledge and then added so much of his own that a comprehensive theory and body of information was available to people interested in personality from diverse points of view. At the time of *Explorations*, the zeitgeists in the field of personality had advanced to a level where they had certain demands that only a work like *Explorations* could fulfill.

The zeitgeists demanded case studies and biographies as well as empirical and experimental work with quantification. *Explorations* met these demands. The zeitgeist for personality theorists accepted the importance of the unconscious, but they also wanted more than that. Many American psychologists interested in personality were becoming increasingly aware of the importance of the conscious aspects of behavior. *Explorations* views behavior as multidimensional and as having multilevels, so conscious, preconscious, and unconscious data are all dealt with and integrated. There was a readiness to accept supplementing theoretical abstractions with well-defined variables that could be studied and experimentally manipulated. *Explorations* provides a comprehensive classification of personality needs. But it does not stop there. Congruent with the emphasis on the environment by the American zeitgeists, *Explorations* provides a most comprehensive classification of variables for the study of environments— the definitions of *press*.

American psychology was also ready for more than studies of abnormal and mentally ill patients for the understanding of all human behavior. What could be more fulfilling than *Explorations,* which provides a comprehensive work devoted to a study of Harvard students who provided *prima facie* evidence of being psychologically healthy individuals? It was now certain that studies of abnormal and mentally ill patients that focus primarily on the catabolic characteristics of personality are not sufficient for the understanding of human behavior.

Conclusion

Explorations had many important effects on clinical assessment and personality research. As one of the most important, it provided invaluable stimulation and support for the TAT. The TAT may have been initiated by suggestions from Morgan; it may have been suggested by a graduate student; or it might have been some other event that impinged itself on Murray's consciousness. Whatever may have been the initial stimulus, the fact remains that without Murray's initiative and support, it would never have developed into the valuable test it became. The story as it unfolds in this area is not too different from what frequently occurs in other creative endeavors, where it is also a question of who should get credit for a creative work, the person who comes up with the idea, the person who develops it, or both. Insofar as the TAT is concerned, there are many credible initial sources, but the fact that it developed and survived is no doubt attributable primarily to Murray.

References

Bartlett, J. (1980). *Familiar quotations: A collection of passages, phrases and proverbs traced to their sources in ancient and modern literature.* Boston, MA: Little, Brown.

Brittain, H. L. (1907). A study in imagination. *Pedagogical Seminary, 14,* 137–207.

Clark, L. P. (1926). The phantasy method of analyzing narcissistic neuroses. *Medical Journal Review, 123,* 154–158.

Jung, C. G. (1973). Studies in word association. In H. Read, M. Fordham, G. Adler, & W. McGuirl (Eds.), *The collected works of C. G. Jung. Vol. 2: Experimental researches* (Bollengin Series XX, Pt. I, pp. 1–480). Princeton, NJ: Princeton University Press. (Original work published 1904–1919)

Libby, W. (1908). The imagination of adolescents. *American Journal of Psychology, 19,* 249–252.

Morgan, C. D., & Murray, H. A. (1935). A method of investigating fantasies: The Thematic Apperception Test. *Archives of Neurology and Psychiatry, 34,* 289–306.

Murray, H. A. (Ed.). (1938). *Explorations in personality: A clinical and experimental study of fifty men of college age.* New York: Oxford University Press.

Murray, H. A. (1967). Henry A. Murray: The case of Murr. In E. T. Boring & G. Lindzey (Eds.), *A history of psychology and autobiography* (pp. 283–310). New York: Appleton-Century-Crofts.

Murstein, B. I. (1963). *Theory and research in projective techniques (emphasizing the TAT).* New York: Wiley.

Robinson, F. G. (1992). *Love's story told: A life of Henry A. Murray.* Cambridge, MA: Harvard University Press.

Schwartz, C. A. (1932). Social-situations pictures in the psychiatric interview. *American Journal of Orthopsychiatry, 2,* 124–133.

Tomkins, S. S. (1947). *The Thematic Apperception Test: The theory and technique of interpretation.* New York: Grune & Stratton.

Triplet, R. G. (1992). Harvard psychology, the Psychological Clinic, and Henry A. Murray: A case study in the establishment of disciplinary boundaries. In C. A. Elliott & N. W. Rossiter (Eds.), *Science at Harvard: Historical perspectives.* Bethlehem, PA: Lehigh University Press.

3

Henry A. Murray and the Creation of the Thematic Apperception Test

James William Anderson

In a book exploring the Thematic Apperception Test (TAT), the most desirable chapter would be an account by Henry A. Murray of his experiences with the development of the test. Murray, who died in 1988, never wrote such an account. But fortunately I interviewed him on just this subject. In addition to two formal interviews, in 1973 at the very beginning of my 15-year friendship with him, I discussed the TAT with him several other times. He also gave me copies of several unpublished papers related to the TAT and projection. Drawing on my interviews as well as published and unpublished works, I attempt in this chapter to reconstruct how he came to create and then to refine the TAT—along with the help of his coworkers at the Harvard Psychological Clinic—how he viewed this highly influential test, and what he thought about the way others used the test.

Murray's "Rebirth"

To understand what the TAT meant to Murray, it is necessary to know about what he once called his "rebirth": the dramatic change in his life that brought him to psychology (Harvard College Class of 1915, 1965, p. 367).

His actual birth took place in 1893. His family was part of the tiny segment who stood at the top of New York society. He had what he jokingly called the childhood of "an average, privileged American boy" (Murray, 1967, p. 298)—the humor stems from the wide gap between the life of an average boy and an average privileged boy. His family lived in a New York brownstone and summered at Wave Crest on Long Island, where they built a home so lavish that Murray was embarrassed even among his friends who also belonged to wealthy families (Murray interview, October 3, 1987). Murray graduated from the Groton School and Harvard University—the same institutions Franklin D. Roosevelt attended a few years earlier.

Murray then went on to medical school at Columbia University. After receiving his MD in 1919, he did further work at Columbia in biology and received his MA in 1920. Murray felt that he experienced his early years as if he were sleep walking. He had little awareness of his inner world or his surroundings. He went through life "as if it were a play"; he started to wake up when he was in medical school (Murray interview, October 2, 1987).

After a surgical internship, he turned his attention to laboratory research. Focusing on the development of chicken embryos, he worked for 4 years at the Rockefeller Institute in New York City and then continued his research at Cambridge University, where he eventually received a PhD in biochemistry in 1927. As a laboratory scientist, he published 21 articles (Anderson, 1990).

But during the latter part of this period, he underwent what he described as a "profound affectional upheaval" (Murray, 1967, p. 290). Central to his transformation was his discovery of the inner world. Previously, he had seen the individual as something similar to a robot. After developing his new view, when he looked at a person, Murray (1940) visualized

> a flow of powerful subjective life, conscious and unconscious; a whispering gallery in which voices echo from the distant past; a gulf stream of fantasies with floating memories of past events, currents of contending complexes, plots and counterplots, hopeful intimations and ideals. (p. 160)

His engagement with great works of art helped show him that there was a transcendent realm of which he had been largely ignorant. He was moved by the music of Beethoven, Wagner, and Puccini. The philosophical writings of Nietzsche, the plays of Eugene O'Neill, and the novels of Dostoyevsky, Proust, and Hardy were among the works to which he was exposed (Murray, 1967, pp. 290, 293). Most fateful, though, was his discovery of Melville, with whom he came to have a life-long fascination. On first reading *Moby-Dick,* he was "swept by Melville's gale and shaken by his appalling sea dragon" (Murray, 1951/1981, p. 83).

Soon he learned that there was a discipline, psychodynamic psychology, that deals with this realm. A first, exciting encounter with Carl Jung's (1923) *Psychological Types* "led to an omnivorous and nourishing process of readings through the revolutionary and astonishing works of Sigmund Freud and his disciples, heady liquor for the young chemist" (Murray, 1967, p. 289).

Although not unhappily married, Murray fell in love with a woman who shared and played a central role in inspiring his new interests. Christiana Drummond Morgan, who was also married, was an artist who had been taken with Jungian psychology. Someone with unusual intuition and artistic sensitivity, she was at home in the world with which Murray was just becoming acquainted. At C. Morgan's suggestion, Murray visited Jung in 1925 "supposedly to discuss abstractions; but in a day or two to my astonishment enough affective stuff erupted to invalid a pure scientist" (Murray, 1940, p. 153).

Murray soon decided to make a radical change in both his professional and personal lives. Although well on his way to a successful career in biochemistry, he abandoned that field and turned to psychology (Anderson, 1988). Also although neither of them got divorced, he and C. Morgan began an intimate emotional, intellectual, and sexual relationship that lasted until her death in 1967.

Murray's Approach to Psychology

Through a series of improbable circumstances, Murray became first an assistant at the Harvard Psychological Clinic and then, 2 years later in 1929, director of the clinic and an assistant professor of psychology (Robinson, 1992). Murray had turned his life upside down because of a burning desire to study the inner world. When he discovered what academic psychology was like, he was not just disappointed but disgusted. "I didn't have any respect for the psychology that was taught and for the people who taught it. . . . They had trained incapacity. They were trained to have tunnel vision" (Murray interview, June 18, 1976). Murray believed that psychologists were preoccupied with trying to prove that they were scientists. Having already demonstrated his skill as a scientist, he cared little for that goal. The rewards went to those who could use "the most reliable and precise methods" (Murray, 1967, p. 293). As a result, psychologists were drawn to studying trivial aspects of organisms. The most unruly area, "the darker, blinder recesses of the psyche," was "anathema" (p. 293) to most psychologists.

Murray (1940) thought psychologists should try to understand

> why man, "like an angry ape, plays such fantastic tricks before high heaven," why he laughs, blasphemes and frets, cheers at a spangled cloth and bleeds for a king; why he blushes over four-letter words and hides his genitals, and falls in love with so and so and later strangles her; why he mourns in isolation, lacerates himself with guilt, invents a purgatory and a paradise. (p. 150)

Instead, he found the leading journals filled with such articles as "The Effects of the Direction of Initial Pathways on the Orientation of White Mice in a Maze" (Ebersbach & Washburn, 1930) and "Apparatus for Studying Eyelid Responses" (Allison, 1930). He described the elaborate procedures of experimental psychologists as "a mountain of ritual bringing forth a mouse of fact more dead than alive" (Murray, 1967, p. 305). Never one to keep his opinions to himself, he published his view early in his career that

> academic psychology has contributed practically nothing to the knowledge of human nature. It has not only failed to bring light to the great, hauntingly recurrent problems, but it has no intention, one is shocked to realize, of attempting to investigate them. (Murray, 1935/1981, p. 339)

The Setting for the Creation of the
Thematic Apperception Test

Murray believed that academic psychology had languished because it concentrated on the phenomena, such as eyelid responses, that were easiest to investigate, despite their unimportance. His conviction that psychologists should study the "darker, blinder" strata left him with a quandary. How could one get at the most hidden aspects of the psyche?

He told me that he had long had an interest in projection for just this reason. He noticed that in primitive religions, people endow "objects of awe" with qualities characteristic of the human mind. The object might be seen as having a feeling or an aim that would be to the worshiper's benefit or detriment. The worshiper might, for example, ascribe meaning to a "great black cloud or hear God's voice in a hurricane" (Murray interview, May 23, 1973). But the cloud or the hurricane is an inanimate object. The worshiper's depiction of it reflects something coming from the worshiper's psyche. Projection is "the best way of learning about somebody next to his being aware and anxious to tell you" (Murray interview, May 23, 1973).

Murray was well aware that he was not thinking of projection in Freud's sense of the term (Murray, circa 1950s). Freud defined *projection* (in German *projektion*) as a defense mechanism that worked in a specific way. The individual has an unacceptable feeling or wish and gains some relief from it by attributing it to someone else: "The proposition 'I hate him' becomes transformed by projection into another one: 'He hates (persecutes) me, which will justify me in hating him' " (Freud, 1911/1958, p. 63). In the early 1930s, Murray already saw projection as a more general process that was not necessarily defensive. He realized that individuals draw on their own inner world in imagining the characteristics of people or objects around them.

The first psychological experiment Murray (1933/1981) conducted involved projection. His participants, all 11 years old, were his daughter, Josephine, and four of her friends who were staying overnight at the Murray house. The experiment must have been conducted in 1932 because that was the year Josephine was 11 years old. Murray had the girls rate a set of photographs of faces on the basis of how good or bad they thought the person was, whether kind and loving or cruel and malicious. Ratings were conducted in the afternoon, repeated after they had played a frightening game called Murder in the darkened house, and conducted again the next day. As expected, the ratings made after the game were significantly different in the direction of maliciousness than the ratings made at the two other times. The pictures were the same, but the girls saw them as being more malicious because of the fear that the game had precipitated in them.

One error Murray made that weakened his results was using his daughter as a participant. She did not rate the faces as being more malicious after the game. Murray thought the main reason was that she was used to the house and therefore did not find the game as scary as the others did (Murray interview, May 23, 1973).

In the article on this experiment, Murray discussed two processes, apperception and projection, that were also central to the TAT. He differentiated apperception, a term which he said had been defined by C. F. Stout, from perception. *Perception,* he wrote, refers to recognition based on sensory impressions; *apperception* refers to the process by which additional meaning is assigned to the object (Murray, 1933/1981, p. 275). His experiment was an attempt to demonstrate apperception, in that the additional maliciousness the girls saw in the photographs after playing Murder was something that the girls assigned to the photographs.

Murray (1933/1981) defined projection as "the process whereby psychic elements—needs, feelings and emotions, or images and contexts of images activated by such affective states—are referred by the experiencing subject to the external world without sufficient objective evidence" (p. 277). In putting the two processes together, Murray coined the term "apperceptive projection."[1]

Meanwhile, with a determination to explore personality in depth, Murray developed an investigative approach that was radically different from anything else in psychology. He first used this approach with a group of participants in 1932 (Triplet, 1983, p. 187). The approach consisted of a number of investigators studying the same group of participants over a substantial period of time. Murray and his coworkers at the Harvard Psychological Clinic were looking for different methods and experimental procedures to use for studying the participants.

Discovery of the Thematic Apperception Test

After his experiment on maliciousness, Murray (interview, May 23, 1973) told me, "I got around to the point where I thought it wasn't enough to know about one variable"; he began looking at fantasies. According to Murray's account, a student of his named Cecelia Washburn Roberts was curious about what blind people meant by words such as *see*. She was interested in comparing their fantasies with those of people with sight. She tried to get her son to tell her his fantasies, but probably because he was ill with a cold, he was not very cooperative. She had a child's book nearby and asked him to tell her a story about one of the pictures; he then created a rich fantasy. She told Murray about this experience. Murray recalled that the idea behind the TAT "came specifically in my mind when she told the story of her son" (Murray interview, May 23, 1973).[2]

By the time Murray had his conversation with Roberts (Murray interview, December 31, 1973), he had already been collecting pictures to use projection in the study of personality. Participants were asked, What's

---

[1]Editor's note: In the early 1930s, Murray also supervised research on apperception by one of his students, Nevitt Sanford. The results were later reported in two articles (Sanford, 1936, 1937).

[2]Editor's note: It is difficult to date Murray's conversation with Roberts. Murray (interview, December 31, 1973) thought it was probably in 1933 because he remembered it as taking place after the experiment on maliciousness, which was conducted in 1932. He also said that he talked with Roberts a short time before he tried the procedure with his mother in early 1934. Roberts took a year-long course with Murray in 1930–1931, but she continued taking other courses in psychological research in the 1931–1932 and 1932–1933 academic years (D. G. Winter, personal communication, August 1996), so she might have had the conversation with Murray in 1933, as he recalled. One contradictory piece of evidence is that Nevitt Sanford recalled that work on the TAT began earlier in the 1930s (see Gieser & W. Morgan, chap. 5, this volume). Chronologies of events at the clinic by Douglas (1993) and Robinson (1992) seem to be consistent with this recollection.

in the picture? But what interested Murray the most was apperception, that is, What is beyond the picture? He found that most of the participants said the same things, but that "didn't tell me enough" (Murray interview, May 23, 1973). The turning point came when participants were "asked to imagine something, to get away from the facts"; once the directions "turned to the imaginative" (Murray interview, May 23, 1973), the TAT was born.

Murray related to me that he immediately received "confirmation" of the value of asking people to tell stories "by choosing pictures and giving them to someone I knew, a lady who had just lost her husband and I knew she was grieving." He added, "the stories were all about herself grieving and her husband. She had no idea these were about herself." He did not mention this confirmation in the original article on the TAT because he "didn't want it to fall in the hands of the woman" (Murray interview, May 23, 1973).

He told me only later that this woman was his mother. After his father's death in the spring of 1934, Murray spent a few days with his mother in the country. He showed her several pictures in an "offhand way" and asked her to tell him some stories. "She didn't think it was a test," he recalled. "I felt a little bashful about showing them at all; she didn't realize she was giving [her feelings] away" (Murray interview, December 31, 1973). At the time, his mother was numb and could not understand why she had so little emotion. Her stories "were almost as gross as this, 'This woman has lost her husband' " (Murray interview, July 31, 1980); they also included the feelings with which she was out of touch. Murray almost would have thought she had been teasing him, except that would have been totally out of character for her. Her stories were so revealing that Murray felt "guilty."

One could hardly imagine a more dramatic demonstration of the power of an experimental procedure. The thematic apperception method caused his very own mother not only to communicate feelings that she did not intend to share with her son but also to express feelings from which she had been blocked off. "When [a procedure] works, it works," he noted, "and [it] tells you something you didn't get any other way" (Murray interview, December 31, 1973).

A short time later, he showed his daughter, Josephine, a picture of an older man who looked angry. "This man is trying to write a book," she said. "He is angry because it isn't going better. She described," Murray concluded, "just how I felt every day." (He was struggling at the time to write *Explorations in Personality* [Robinson, 1992, p. 217].) Murray saw these two demonstrations as the best way of checking on the validity of a procedure. Because he knew his mother and his daughter, he felt certain that the method of having people tell stories, prompted by pictures, revealed something about their inner worlds. A later step, he added, would be to try correlations, with experimental participants, between the results of the procedure and other information that has been gathered on the participants (Murray interview, July 31, 1980).

One of the early experiences that "sold" Murray on the TAT involved a young man who had come to the hospital with a minor illness. "I'm not worried about that," the man's father said to the doctor, "but he's lost three jobs because they believe he's stolen something" (Murray interview, December 31, 1973). The father did not think his son was guilty but asked the doctor to question him about it. The doctor asked the young man but with no success. The young man then took the TAT. As Murray recalled, "it all became quite apparent: that he was interested in stealing. Also the motive; he was stealing to impress the girl he was in love with." The young man had a "complacent manner" and "didn't feel he had revealed anything" (Murray interview, May 23, 1973). But when he was shown the stories, he admitted what he had done (see also Murray, 1936/1981, p. 379).

When looking at the discovery of the idea behind the TAT, Murray focused on the conversation he had with Roberts in which she told him about the story her son had made up; there are at least three other influences that are likely to have played a part.

First, Murray was well aware that novels and short stories often, perhaps always, reflect the inner world of the author. As he explained it in the original article on the TAT, "another fact which was relied on in devising the present method is that a great deal of written fiction is the conscious or unconscious expression of the author's experiences or fantasies" (C. Morgan & Murray, 1935, p. 289). Murray knew from his reading that many psychological thinkers, including Freud, had commented on this fact. The specific influence—most likely an unconscious influence— of a scene in one of Thomas Wolfe's novels, as hypothesized by Gieser and W. Morgan (see chap. 5, this volume), cannot be excluded.

Second, Murray was familiar with the Rorschach test. The original article on the TAT notes that projection "is utilized in the Rorschach test" (C. Morgan & Murray, 1935, p. 289), and the Rorschach was included among the procedures used in the research reported in *Explorations in Personality* (Murray, 1938, p. 582). Even though the Rorschach test and the TAT both rely on projection, there is a major difference. In the Rorschach, participants report on the forms they see when they look at inkblots. The distinguishing feature of the TAT is that it involves making up dramatic stories, and that activity has no counterpart on the Rorschach test.

Third, Murray knew about Jung's method of induced visions, also called "active imagination." Murray described this method, in an article published just a year after the article that introduced the TAT. This method involves instructing the participant "to concentrate intensely upon the first image that arises distinctly in his mind [and then] to visualize this image or scene with greater and greater clarity" (Murray, 1936/1981, p. 375).

C. Morgan was the main source of Murray's familiarity with the method of induced visions. In Zurich, Switzerland, Jung taught C. Morgan this method during her psychotherapy with him in 1925 and showed her pictures he had made of his own visions. Returning to the United States in 1927, she continued the practice of visioning and painted a series of watercolors that depicted her visions. She sent these paintings to Jung with verbal descriptions of the visions. He was enthusiastic about her material and said he often thought of working through this material. From 1930 to 1934, he presented a series of 13 seminars in which he examined her visions as a way of illustrating his psychological approach (Murray, 1976).

Whereas Jung built a series of seminars around C. Morgan's visions, Murray, if anything, was even more fascinated by them. At times, he believed that he and C. Morgan should use her visions, which he called "trances," as the central guiding force in their lives. "It is my complete conviction," he once wrote to her, "that these trances of yours must be worked over, and lived, and merged into our life, so that they are the reality and the essence of our tangible existence" (Douglas, 1993, p. 304).

A vision that C. Morgan produced in this way has much in common with a TAT story; both may be considered fantasies. In addition, C. Morgan's visions are linked to pictures, as is also true with TAT stories. The difference, though, is that she used her paintings to help express her fantasies, whereas in the case of the TAT stories, the participant is shown a picture as a spur to making up a fantasy.[3]

Development of the Thematic Apperception Test

The Harvard Psychological Clinic provided the ideal setting for the development of the TAT. A group of participants was available for experiments. In addition, as the director, Murray could draw on a substantial number of colleagues to help him with his work.

Murray quickly saw the advantages of having a set of pictures that could be given to a variety of participants. The next task was to develop this set of pictures. Murray commented on five factors that played a part in the choice of the pictures that were used.

1. An attempt was made for the set of pictures to be *comprehensive*. A picture was chosen to suggest a "critical situation" and to evoke a "fantasy related to it." In the article that introduced the TAT, C. Morgan and Murray (1935) noted that "ideally, there should be a picture which would act as a trellis to support the growth and unfolding of every root fantasy" (p. 290). For example, in the current set of cards, a picture shows a man with an older woman and another picture shows a man with an older man. (These are among the cards used with male participants.) TAT commentators pointed out that these pictures often elicit stories reflecting participants' feelings regarding parental figures (Henry, 1956, pp. 246–248).

2. *Ambiguity* was taken into account in choosing the pictures (Murray, 1943, p. 1). Murray found that he tended at first to pick pic-

---

[3]Editor's note: Some of C. Morgan's drawings and paintings appear in Douglas (1997).

tures that "told too much," in other words, that would elicit the same general storyline from most participants. He realized it was a problem when "too much was settled in the nature of the picture" (Murray interview, October 2, 1987). Participants had to be given room to create stories that reflected their inner worlds.

Card 3 BM in the current series of TAT cards shows a person on the floor and leaning against a couch. Murray told me that after he came across a particular photograph of a boy, "I showed it to people, and some said, 'a boy,' and some said, 'a girl.' I immediately picked it for that reason." C. Morgan redrew the picture to make the gender of the figure even more indeterminate (Murray interview, October 2, 1987). In a later study with 50 male participants, 44% saw the figure as a boy, 50% saw the figure as a girl, and 6% were uncertain (Rosenzweig, 1949, p. 489). The image near the boy, which might be a gun, a knife, or a set of keys, was also drawn to look ambiguous (Murray interview, October 2, 1987). One of Murray's favorite TAT pictures was Card 14, which shows the silhouette of a person against a window; the reason he liked this picture so well is that "it's so ambiguous" (Murray interview, October 2, 1987).

3. Another initial consideration was "that there should be at least one person in each picture with whom the subject could easily *identify* himself" (emphasis added; C. Morgan & Murray, 1935, p. 290). For that reason, in the current series of cards, there are somewhat varying sets of cards for use with men, women, boys, and girls.[4]

    Murray pointed out that the term *identification* could be confusing because it usually refers to the process of putting oneself in the position of another. In connection with the TAT, it refers to

> a process whereby a story-teller feels or imagines himself *inside* a character he is *creating* (rather than looking at the character from the outside) and thus gets into a relationship with his character which is similar (inside, close, intimate) to the relationship that he has with his own psyche. (Murray, circa 1961)[5]

4. The overriding principle was to determine which pictures had the greatest "*stimulating power*" (emphasis added; Murray, 1943, p. 2). Murray (interview, May 23, 1973) had already collected thousands of pictures for conducting experiments with projection. In developing the first set of 20 pictures, he and his colleagues used a larger number of pictures and assessed how effective each one was at evoking stories that illuminated the central features of the participants' personalities (C. Morgan & Murray, 1935, p. 290). It was possible to make this evaluation because the yield from the stories could be compared with the voluminous information that had been gathered on the participants from the many

---

[4]The current series of cards also include three cards without any people: Card 12 BG, Card 16 (Blank card), and Card 19 (see W. G. Morgan, chap. 6, this volume).

[5]This 4-page paper was written in 1961 or 1962.

other investigations of them conducted at the clinic.

Many of the pictures were redrawn versions of photographs or paintings. One example is Card 3 BM, described above. Another example is Card 1, showing a boy with a violin, which is based on a photograph of Yehudi Menuhin (Murray interview, October 2, 1987; see also Jahnke & Morgan, 1997). According to the TAT manual, six cards were drawn or redrawn by C. Morgan and nine pictures were drawn or redrawn by Samuel Thal. W. Morgan (see chap. 6, this volume) gives more detailed information on the origins of the TAT images.

The principle of finding the most productive pictures took precedence over the principle of having an obvious identificatory figure in each picture (Murray, 1943, p. 2). For example, Card 1, which depicts a boy, is used with female as well as male participants. Cards 12 BG, 16, and 19 have no people in them at all.

5. One additional principle, of which Murray was not aware, influenced him in the choice of pictures. Certain pictures appealed to him because of his own personality. Often I have had participants remark that the cards are depressing and that many of them seem to pull for distressing stories. Murray agreed with me when I suggested that his own depressive tendency had an impact on the pictures in the TAT (Murray interview, October 2, 1987). On another occasion, he referred to his "marrow of misery and melancholy" (Murray, 1967, p. 299). He told me that he saw an advantage to having pictures like these because such pictures elicit stories "of abnormal states of existence" (Murray interview, October 2, 1987). An "everyday picture," he said, leads to less of a story. He acknowledged that he is "drawn to sad stories." He noted that the tragedies of Shakespeare appeal to him more than the comedies. He said that his favorite opera is *Tosca*. "That ends in suicide; it's a sad one." He also told me that his favorite TAT card is 3 BM, which shows a figure huddling on the floor and has probably the most depressive cast of any of the cards.

People who are familiar with Murray might be surprised that he ever settled on a final series of TAT cards; he was notorious for not completing projects, and he was continually overflowing with new ideas. In fact, he commented to me, "we [he and his colleagues] would have gone on changing the pictures if the war hadn't come up" (Murray interview, December 31, 1973). Apparently, when he left Harvard in 1943 to lead the assessment program of the Office of Strategic Services, he decided to publish the test in the state that it was in at that time.

Just as it was out of character for Murray to settle on a final version of the TAT, it would have been out of character for him to stop with one way of administering the test. The TAT manual provides a standardized approach (Murray, 1943, pp. 3–5): The tester gives instructions, which emphasize that the participant is to make up a story for each picture, and then presents the participant with a set of 20 cards. Later, TAT specialists have made minor modifications in administration; for example, Rapaport, Gill, and Schafer

(1968, pp. 469–470) provided different instructions and had the participant facing the tester rather than with his or her back to the tester, as the manual suggests.

Murray and his colleagues continually thought about and experimented with different ways of administering the test. Murray (interview, October 3, 1987) recalled, for example, that Silvan Tomkins once gave a single picture to a participant each morning for several days to see how the stories would vary. Other variations were to ask the participant to "tell a funny story," "tell a child's story that you'd tell a child," or "imagine yourself a child and tell a story as a child would at the age of six" (Murray interview, December 31, 1973). Instead of asking for one detailed story to a card, Murray (1951) and his colleagues asked the participant "to respond to each picture by presenting the outline of as many plots as possible" (p. 578).

Role of C. Morgan in the Development of the Test

A vexing question, probably impossible to answer definitively, is the role of C. Morgan in the development of the TAT. The authorship of the original article announcing the creation of the TAT was given as C. Morgan and Murray (1935). The section of *Explorations in Personality* (Murray, 1938) that describes the TAT is an amended version of the earlier article and is ascribed to C. Morgan and Murray. The authorship of an early TAT manual does not include C. Morgan's name (White, Sanford, Murray, & Bellak, 1941), but the title of the manual is the *Morgan–Murray Thematic Apperception Test*. The manual of the published version of the test—the version still in use today—refers to the test as the "Thematic Apperception Test," the full authorship of the manual is listed as Murray and Staff of the Harvard Psychological Clinic (1943).

In 1985, after Edwin Shneidman referred to Murray in a publication of Radcliffe College as the developer of the TAT, an alumna named Dorothy Tobkin wrote a letter noting that C. Morgan coauthored the test. Tobkin (1985) added angrily, "as women, we should not, as men too often have done, let [outstanding women] remain unrecognized" (p. 2).

Murray (1985) replied with

> the word "author" in this connection is susceptible to several distinct references, one of which is this: the germinal suggestion for the TAT came not from [C.] Morgan but from an unusually apperceptive student in abnormal psychology at Radcliffe, Mrs. Cecelia Roberts. . . . The next phase in the development of the TAT involved the choice of pictures and testing a variety of modes of administration. It was at this point that Christiana Morgan had the main role. When the first article announcing the new method was written, her name was placed first, but when she found that the ensuing mail was consequently all directed to her, she asked that her name be officially omitted thereafter. (p. 2)

In an earlier article, he presented a similar description of the roles of Roberts and C. Morgan (Murray, 1951, p. 577).

But in communications with me, he gave a somewhat different version of this matter. "She didn't want her name on the paper," he told me. Letters came addressed to her because she was listed as the first author. "She didn't want to answer them and couldn't," he added. "She gave them to me." I asked him why he had put her name first on the original TAT article. "To get her interested," Murray replied; "I wanted some help in starting it" (Murray interview, January 1, 1987).

"She wasn't specially interested in that kind of thing," he told me another time. He said that as a Jungian analyst, "she was interested like other analysts in questions having to do with therapy but not so much with investigations and especially tests" (Murray interview, October 2, 1987).

Stirred up by our discussions on this topic, he wrote me a letter. It said the following in part:

> At the last meeting, the topic was Christiana Morgan and her influence on my life and work. . . . It was her general judgment on matters of development which were decisive for me and not any details in regard to scientific tests of any sort. She was there in the beginning of the enterprise but took no interest in the results of the experiments. Her main social function was depth psychotherapy. She understood many things that baffled others. Several writings in her name were published by me.[6]

C. Morgan's biographer, Claire Douglas (1993, pp. 203–206, 350), argued that the TAT was perhaps C. Morgan's "most original contribution" and that she deserved to be listed as its first author. Two psychologists who were involved in the clinic at the time, Saul Rosenzweig and Robert White, remembered that C. Morgan was centrally involved with the test. Douglas located notes in which C. Morgan wrote about the TAT, and she cited a 14-page manuscript in which C. Morgan explored the concept of the "claustrum" in part as it relates to TAT responses. Yet Douglas (1993) also quoted a manuscript Murray wrote in 1940. Speaking in the third person, Murray (in Douglas, 1993) noted that "she had influenced him to push the work at the Clinic more and more from the old mechanical experiments, until he finally devised for her use the Thematic Apperception Test, his one contribution to methodology" (pp. 268–269).

In 1949, he publicly assigned a secondary role to C. Morgan in a brief account of the history of the TAT. He said she helped find pictures, redrew some of them, and did some of the administration of the test to the participants; he added that they had written the initial TAT article together (Holt, 1949).[7]

---

[6]This undated letter to me was never mailed. Eugene Taylor, who worked as Murray's research assistant, gave me a copy of this letter.

[7]Editor's note: Both of C. Morgan's parents died in 1933, and her husband died in 1934. According to Caroline C. Murray (personal communication, September 13, 1997), Harry Murray told her that he helped C. Morgan through her grief, including guilt about their extramarital affair, by encouraging her involvement in the clinic. H. Murray added that this encouragement culminated in his giving C. Morgan first authorship of the article that introduced the TAT.

As I see it, the TAT grew out of Murray's entire history up to that time in his life. He gave up a promising career as a researcher in the hard sciences and devoted the rest of his life to psychology. C. Morgan played a central role, not only in his interest in psychology but also in his emphasis on the depths of the psyche, which he described as "a land of mysterious formations" (Murray, 1938, p. 729). Although C. Morgan was not specifically interested in the TAT, she was, as he told me, "interested in everything I was doing" (Murray interview, October 2, 1987). He shared all his thinking, passions, and struggles with her. She no doubt had a part in every step of the work on the TAT: gathering and choosing pictures, drawing several of the pictures herself, and administering the test. But many other people at the Harvard Psychological Clinic also participated in these activities, such as Nevitt Sanford, Frederic Wyatt, Jurgen Ruesch, and Samuel Thal. Thal drew more of the pictures in the final TAT series than C. Morgan did (Murray, 1943, pp. 18–19).

Still, in one sense, the TAT was a collaboration between Murray and C. Morgan. As Murray noted in the 1940 manuscript mentioned above, when he met C. Morgan, he approached "everything with his intellect, naming, classifying, cataloging" (Douglas, 1993, p. 267). C. Morgan was largely responsible for his undergoing "a long series of conversions" (p. 270) in the direction of his involvement with the realm of feeling and imagination. The TAT, even if primarily Murray's creation, was a product of his attempt to combine the two sides of his personality. In the TAT, Murray's intellectual, analytical skills were integrated with his interest in fantasy—an interest that developed in tandem with his relationship with C. Morgan.

Murray's Observations on the Use of the Test

Once, I asked Murray for his reactions to a small research project, involving the TAT, that I was conducting. I was looking at the TAT protocols of two groups of adolescents. On the basis of other material, they had been characterized as the "tumultuous-growth" group and the "consistent-growth" group. Murray had a negative reaction to this research. He did not see much value in sorting the adolescents into these two large divisions. He commented that

> now I see that all generalizations like that are out for human beings—that is, that there is so much diversity, and the diversity depends on so many different factors . . . that you can't make these big groupings. (Murray interview, August 19, 1975)

I pointed out that using certain previously developed measures of conflict, I had found some statistically significant differences between the TAT protocols of the two groups, with more conflict in the tumultuous-growth group and less in the consistent-growth group. In what I now see as a typical comment from him, he stated the following:

> I would be interested in the ones that were put in the tumultuous group but didn't show an unusual amount of conflict and [the conflicts in] those that were put in the nice quiet group, . . . the consistent group. [I would be interested in] the boy in school, the adolescent that's so well behaved, and the teacher said, "He's one of my best pupils. He's good as gold. He hardly says anything. He never breaks any rules." And then he all of a sudden shoots his father or something. (Murray interview, August 19, 1975)

His interest was in getting at the individuality of each person, and he believed that much research glossed over and lost that individuality.

On another occasion, I asked Murray what he thought of the various ways the TAT had been used. At first, he was hesitant to make any criticisms. "It wasn't meant to be restricted to any one conceptual school," Murray (interview, May 23, 1973) noted, and he was pleased that so many chapters and articles had been written which made use of the test.

But it was not in character for him to hold back his opinions, and soon they started tumbling out. He concentrated on the way the test was administered. His underlying point, though, was that testers did not have enough respect for the TAT's potential power. "They run through six or eight cards in 50 minutes and let it go at that," Murray (interview, May 23, 1973) commented. He preferred to have the whole test given, 20 cards in 2 sessions of 1 hour each.

He also felt that many psychologists did not give the directions in a way that encouraged the participant to talk freely. He thought that emphasis should be put on "dramatic imagination." If the participant has not gotten the idea after the first story, the tester should "repeat the directions with a proper emphasis on literary imagination" (Murray interview, May 23, 1973). He thought that as a rule, if the participant did not make up stories of at least 250 words, then the directions had not been given correctly.

Murray's most strongly felt complaint was that many people did not appreciate the capacity of the TAT to give them access to the inner world. "My idea," he said, "was to illuminate the unconscious processes—that were repressed—of which the subject was not aware. That was the whole point of it" (Murray interview, May 23, 1973). He pointed out that he and Gordon Allport often disagreed because Allport believed that if you wanted to learn something about someone, you should merely ask the person about it (Murray, 1958, pp. 188–189). But Murray superintended the creation of the TAT precisely because it helped bring out that about which one cannot learn by asking directly. He summarized the purpose of the TAT as

> to bring out what the subject wouldn't say. Now that might be what . . . he didn't want to say but it was conscious, or what he couldn't say because it was unconscious. [In other words, in one case, he] wouldn't tell you because it was private and he didn't want you to know. [In the other case,] he couldn't tell you because he didn't know himself. (Murray interview, May 23, 1973)

Conclusion

Murray believed that the surface people present to the world hardly hints at the hidden depths within, which are wondrous and complex. When he first became a psychologist, he was repelled by academic psychology and its simplistic, one-dimensional view of the human being. His entire career can be seen as an attempt to reveal the inner world and to make sense of it. He disliked being identified as the person who developed the TAT (Hall, 1968, p. 61) because he felt his work on the TAT was only one small part of his contributions as a psychologist. But the TAT is the perfect embodiment of his approach to psychology. It captures his interest in the inner world. It capitalizes on his belief, also represented in his work on Melville, that imaginative fiction feeds on and illustrates an individual's deepest concerns and conflicts. In addition, the TAT provides a way of making what is concealed manifest and of putting a representation of the inner world on paper, so that it becomes accessible to systematic analysis.

References

Allison, L. W. (1930). Apparatus for studying eyelid responses. *American Journal of Psychology, 42,* 634–635.

Anderson, J. W. (1988). Henry Murray's early career: A psychobiographical exploration. *Journal of Personality, 56,* 139–171.

Anderson, J. W. (1990). The life of Henry A. Murray: 1893–1988. In A. I. Rabin, R. A. Zucker, R. A. Emmons, & S. Frank (Eds.), *Studying persons and lives* (pp. 304–334). New York: Springer.

Douglas, C. (1993). *Translate the darkness: The life of Christiana Morgan.* New York: Simon & Schuster.

Douglas, C. (1997). *Visions: Notes of the seminar given in 1930–1934 by C. G. Jung.* Princeton, NJ: Princeton University Press.

Ebersbach, R., & Washburn, M. F. (1930). The effects of the direction of initial pathways on the orientation of white mice in a maze. *American Journal of Psychology, 42,* 413–414.

Freud, S. (1958). Psycho-analytic notes on an autobiographical account of a case of paranoia (dementia paranoides). In J. Strachey (Ed. & Trans.), *The standard edition of the complete psychological works of Sigmund Freud* (Vol. 12, pp. 9–82). London: Hogarth Press. (Original work published 1911)

Hall, M. H. (1968, September). A conversation with Henry A. Murray. *Psychology Today, 2*(4), 56–63.

Harvard College Class of 1915. (1965). *Fiftieth anniversary report.* Cambridge, MA: Harvard University Printing Office.

Henry, W. E. (1956). *The analysis of fantasy: The thematic apperception technique in the study of personality.* New York: Wiley.

Holt, R. R. (1949, Winter). The TAT Newsletter. *Rorschach Exchange & Journal of Projective Techniques, 13,* 229–232.

Jahnke, J., & Morgan, W. G. (1997). A true TAT story. In W. G. Bringmann, H. E. Lück, R. Miller, & C. E. Early (Eds.), *A pictorial history of psychology* (pp. 376–379). Carol Stream, IL: Quintessence.

Jung, C. G. (1923). *Psychological types.* New York: Harcourt, Brace & World.

Morgan, C. D., & Murray, H. M. (1935). A method for investigating fantasies: The Thematic Apperception Test. *Archives of Neurology and Psychiatry, 34,* 289–306.

Murray, H. A. (Ed.). (1938). *Explorations in personality: A clinical and experimental study of fifty men of college age.* New York: Oxford University Press.

Murray, H. A. (1940). What should psychologists do about psychoanalysis? *Journal of Abnormal and Social Psychology, 35,* 150–175.

Murray, H. A. (1943). *Thematic Apperception Test: Manual.* Cambridge, MA: Harvard University Press.

Murray, H. A. (circa 1950s). *Projection.* Unpublished manuscript.

Murray, H. A. (1951). Uses of the Thematic Apperception Test. *American Journal of Psychiatry, 107,* 577–581.

Murray, H. A. (1958). Drive, time, strategy, measurement, and our way of life. In G. Lindzey (Ed.), *Assessment of human motives* (pp. 183–196). New York: Rinehart.

Murray, H. A. (circa 1961). *A few comments relative to the TAT and to the interpretation of story compositions.* Unpublished manuscript.

Murray, H. A. (1967). The case of Murr. In E. G. Boring & G. Lindzey (Eds.), *A history of psychology in autobiography* (Vol. 5, pp. 285–310). New York: Appleton-Century-Crofts.

Murray, H. A. (1976). Postscript: Morsels of information regarding the extraordinary woman in whose psyche the foregoing visions were begot. In C. G. Jung, *The visions seminars* (Book 2, pp. 517–521). Zurich, Switzerland: Spring.

Murray, H. A. (1981). The effect of fear upon estimates of the maliciousness of other personalities. In E. S. Shneidman (Ed.), *Endeavors in psychology: Selections from the personology of Henry A. Murray* (pp. 275–290). New York: Harper & Row. (Original work published 1933)

Murray, H. A. (1981). Psychology and the university. In E. Shneidman (Ed.), *Endeavors in psychology: Selections from the personology of Henry A. Murray* (pp. 337–351). New York: Harper & Row. (Original work published 1935)

Murray, H. A. (1981). Techniques for the systematic investigation of fantasy. In E. S. Shneidman (Ed.), *Endeavors in psychology: Selections from the personology of Henry A. Murray* (pp. 366–389). New York: Harper & Row. (Original work published 1936)

Murray, H. A. (1981). In nomine diaboli. In E. S. Shneidman (Ed.), *Endeavors in psychology: Selections from the personology of Henry A. Murray* (pp. 82–94). New York: Harper & Row. (Original work published 1951)

Murray, H. A. (1985, February). [Letter]. *Second Century Radcliffe News,* p. 2.

Rapaport, D., Gill, M. M., & Schafer, R. (1968). *Diagnostic psychological testing.* New York: International Universities Press.

Robinson, F. (1992). *Love's story told: A life of Henry A. Murray.* Cambridge, MA: Harvard University Press.

Rosenzweig, S. (1949). Apperceptive norms for the Thematic Apperception Test. *Journal of Personality, 17,* 475–503.

Sanford, N. (1936). The effects of abstinence from food upon imaginal processes: A preliminary experiment. *Journal of Psychology, 2,* 129–136.

Sanford, N. (1937). The effects of abstinence from food upon imaginal processes: A further experiment. *Journal of Psychology, 3,* 145–159.

Tobkin, D. (1985, February). [Letter]. *Second Century Radcliffe News,* p. 2.

Triplet, R. G. (1983). *Henry A. Murray and the Harvard Psychological Clinic, 1926–1938: A struggle to expand the disciplinary boundaries of psychology.* Unpublished doctoral dissertation, University of New Hampshire, Durham.

White, R. W., Sanford, N., Murray, H. A., & Bellak, L. (1941). *Morgan–Murray Thematic Apperception Test: Manual of directions.* Cambridge, MA: Harvard University, Harvard Psychological Clinic.

4

Pioneer Experiences in the Clinical Development of the Thematic Apperception Test

Saul Rosenzweig

The recent biography of Henry A. Murray by Forrest Robinson (1992) might be expected to contain significant information about the construction of the Thematic Apperception Test (TAT), the now famous personality assessment device. The book's title, *Love's Story Told,* makes clear, however, that the author had other objectives in mind—themes more oriented toward the libido itself rather than its sublimated expression. Hence, one searches without success for any substantive account of the construction of the TAT. Others accomplish this purpose much more adequately (see Anderson, chap. 3; Gieser & Morgan, chap. 5; Gieser & Stein, chap. 1; and W. G. Morgan, chap. 6, this volume).

I concentrate here on my investigative work with the TAT during a period of 20 years: at the Harvard Psychological Clinic (HPC; Harvard University, Cambridge, MA), at the Worcester State Mental Hospital (WSH; Worcester, MA), and at the Western State Psychiatric Institute and Clinic (WSPI; Pittsburgh, PA). I begin with my minor part in the construction of the technique at HPC, especially my collaboration with Christiana Morgan. My collaboration with her continued when I moved to WSH. Then, while at WSPI, I compiled the first empirical TAT norms. This work was followed by my designing a systematic method of TAT analysis, namely, the composite portrait method (CPM). It was carried out in conjunction with the teaching of both psychometric and projective methods at the University of Pittsburgh; several students and interns in these courses collaborated in the research. CPM was initially presented in my contemporary book *Psychodiagnosis* (Rosenzweig, 1949b), but a separate monograph or periodical contribution, which had been tentatively planned, did not materialize before I left Pittsburgh for St. Louis.

At the Harvard Psychological Clinic

In my halcyon days at Harvard (1925–1934), I had the good fortune of working fairly closely with Murray, director of the HPC, and his collaborator at the clinic, C. Morgan. The clinic was founded by the Boston psychopathologist Morton Prince, author of *The Dissociation of a Personality* (Prince, 1906), which presented in discursive detail the treatment of a patient called "Sally Beauchamp." In a more recent publication, this case is psychoarchaeologically reconstructed, the patient identified, and her idioverse depicted (Rosenzweig, 1987).

My first connection with HPC was when, as a senior undergraduate, I enrolled in the course Dynamic and Abnormal Psychology, offered by Prince, with the assistance of Murray. By then, I was already engaged on the research and writing for my bachelor's honors thesis, devoted to the voluntaristic philosophers Schopenhauer, Nietzsche, and Bergson, on the one hand; and the psychoanalysts Sigmund Freud, Alfred Adler, and Carl Jung, on the other. My thesis turned out to be the key by which I gained admittance to the restricted enrollment for the course. Early in my graduate work, I served as a research assistant to Murray by gathering illustrations from published books and periodicals intended to help in the development of Murray's system of needs, subsequently published in *Explorations in Personality* (Murray, 1938). I also helped him in the search for biographical information concerning the life and work of Herman Melville, Murray's inspirational companion almost from the start of his interest in personality theory.

During the years 1928–1934, when I was officially associated with HPC, that burgeoning institution was housed, first, on 19 Beaver Street, Cambridge, Massachusetts. In about 2 years, a move was made to 64 Plympton Street, where most of my work was done (1930–1934). In this second location, I occupied an office on the second floor, opposite that of C. Morgan, and had a laboratory in the remodeled attic on the third floor that consisted of a room with a slanted ceiling and an adjoining closet, which I rebuilt for use as an observatory into the lab through a one-way mirror. (This type of psychological observation was, I believe, in a pioneer stage at the time.) On the third floor, next to my laboratory, was the office–workshop of Eleanor Jones.[1]

My acquaintance with C. Morgan began in 1928, with my first glimpse of her at an HPC seminar at the Beaver Street location. About 3 years after I joined the HPC staff and had an office there, C. Morgan helped me with the construction of a historical panorama of psychotherapy: a series of pictures in sepia illustrating the development from Egyptian times to the psychoanalytic methods initiated by Freud. The pictures were framed and covered by glass, arranged in chronological sequence, and mounted on a redwood board (measuring about 10 ft [3.05 m] wide by 4 ft [1.22 m] high). Between the pictures were symbolic figures etched into the redwood background. The pictures were bordered by red. Both the figures and the borders were painted by C. Morgan.

In my assistantship to Murray, I was incidentally involved in the se-

---

[1]Editor's note: Jones was a HPC volunteer who worked on the TAT for awhile and with whom Murray became romantically involved. The effects of the Murray-Jones relationship on C. Morgan and her work at the clinic in the early 1930s is discussed by Robinson (1992).

lection of pictures for the TAT, which he and C. Morgan were then starting to develop. It is likely that C. Morgan's paintings of her visions during therapy with Jung were influential in the development of the TAT (see Douglas, 1997, for examples of Morgan's visions artwork and Jung, 1976). C. Morgan, who later painted a number of the TAT pictures, was the person most fully committed to the technique's development (see Douglas, 1993, pp. 203–205). Secondarily, Jones combed through illustrated magazines seeking to discover candidates for what would eventually become the standard stimulus items in the published version, which was issued in 1943 by the Harvard University Press under the authorship of Murray.

At the Worcester State Hospital: Collaboration With C. Morgan

After leaving HPC, I began work on a research service at WSH. One of my projects was concerned with the TAT and was performed through collaborative correspondence with C. Morgan, beginning in 1934. In that year, I moved from Cambridge to Worcester. The first letter concerning work with the TAT was dated March 21, 1935 and runs as follows:

> Perhaps you will recall the suggestion you made some time last year about trying out the Thematic Apperception Test on some psychotics at the hospital. In view of what you were telling me the other night about the exciting results you have been getting, I should like very much to attempt the thing on one or two patients that I am working with rather intensively at the present time. Do you have a set of the pictures and the instructions that you could lend me for a little while?

This letter was answered by C. Morgan on March 27, 1935 as follows:

> Thank you very much for your letter. Unfortunately, there does not seem to be a set of pictures available, but this spring I am going to see if Houghton Mifflin will publish a set, in which case there ought to be some by about June. I will let you know as soon as we have any. It will be most interesting to try them with your cases.

This communication is interesting for its unique mention of Houghton Mifflin as a possible first publisher of the TAT. But nothing appears to have resulted from this initiative.

On November 8, 1935, I wrote a letter to C. Morgan, which begins as follows:

> I received the set of Thematic Apperception cards in good condition and am already making plans for their use. As soon as the necessary material has accumulated, I will send it to you for analysis. Thank you very much.

Here, it is indicated specifically that C. Morgan sent a set of TAT cards to me that was received early in November 1935.

In the same letter of November 8, 1935, as an agent of the psychology department, I invited C. Morgan to present a paper on the Thematic Apperception Test at a psychology seminar. I stated that by then my colleagues and I might have results from some of the patients, so that

> you will have received the material on a couple of psychotics here at the hospital so that you could include an analysis of these results in your presentation. If you prefer to discuss some other phase of the experimentation at the clinic, exclusively or in addition to the Thematic Apperception Test, that would also be agreeable to us. The date we would like to suggest is Tuesday, January 21, 1936.

One week later on November 13, she wrote to thank me for the invitation. But she declined, stating that

> this winter for various reasons I am not letting myself in for any such activities. However, I would love to see your materials and talk it over with you any time that you want or with anyone who is giving the test. We have collected all that material from our various subjects together with the interpretations and anyone who is interested could come here and see me and read the materials which we have.

A paragraph followed about my research on the psychosexual development of schizophrenia patients. The letter then continued and concluded with the following: "Let's see each other and talk over the Thematic Apperception [Test cards] as soon as you have tried them out. I am eager to know whether they will be of any use to you."

On November 27, I wrote to express my regret and to add

> but, on the other hand, we shall be only too glad to avail ourselves of whatever help you are willing to proffer so that in the near future, when the test has been tried on some of our patients, you may expect to hear from me again.

On December 2, she wrote again: "I hope you will try the test before long. It will be great fun to discuss it with you."

It is of incidental but significant interest that two of the letters exchanged with C. Morgan at this time mentioned the surgical operation (radical sympathectomy) that she underwent in 1943. Because there has been doubt expressed about the date of this operation (see Douglas, 1993, pp. 235–247, 355), the following paragraph in the letter of March 19, 1944, is of particular interest:

> I meant to write to you long before this but I was laid low this fall by this new operation which has just been devised for hypertension. It seems to do the trick but is a terror to go through with and I am just beginning to enter the world of the living again.

One of the significant conclusions that can be drawn from the correspondence between C. Morgan and myself is that she was the major contributor to the construction of the TAT. The evidence for this conclusion includes the following: (a) She is named first in the authorship line of the 1935 basic article (C. D. Morgan & Murray, 1935). (b) In a letter dated March 27, 1935, she indicated that she was taking the initiative in finding a publisher for the TAT. She wrote "this spring I am going to see if Houghton Mifflin will publish a set." (c) She, rather than Murray, was doing the active collaborative research with me. (d) It was C. Morgan, not Murray, who was invited to speak at the psychology department colloquium at WSH. (e) Finally, she was clearly responsible for six of the drawings that constituted the pictures of the 1943 published series. The question remains as to why, in publishing the manual in 1943, C. Morgan was not mentioned by Murray as one of the authors.

As noted above, in 1935 C. Morgan sent me a preliminary set of TAT pictures, with the request that I try out their usefulness in the study of schizophrenia patients. Patient protocols in my files indicate that the technique was used with at least two male patients around this time. Unfortunately the set of TAT cards used in the 1930s with patients at WSH has not survived. However, I do have in my possession a complete set of 28 cards (which I refer to as "Series X") that I apparently obtained from C. Morgan after 1941 but prior to the publication of the manual and pictures in 1943. I presume that Series X dates between the years of 1941 and 1943 because one of the pictures included in the set (which also appears as Card 6GF in 1943) is a picture by H. Rubin. This picture did not appear until 1941 when it appeared in *The Saturday Evening Post* (Murray, 1943).[2]

The pictures included in Series X have been compared with the 1943 published series with the conclusion that eight of them are different from the 1943 set. But because these cards were evidently candidates for publication, it may prove useful to describe the relationship between the pictures in the two series. Series X consisted of 28 cards, including 1 blank card. Of these 28, 20 are among the 31 pictures published in 1943. They are as follows (an asterisk indicates that the picture as it appeared in Series X was modified in some way by 1943): 1, 2, 3 BM, *3 GF, *4, *6 BM, *6 GF, *7 BM, 7 GF, *8 BM, 8 GF, *9 BM, 9 GF, *10, 11, *12 M, 14, 15, 16, and 18 BM.

The eight pictures in Series X that were not included in 1943 are described below, numbered as they appeared in Series X.[3] It is possible that C. Morgan, who drew six of the pictures in the published set, drew some of these pictures as well.

---

[2]A detailed study of the vicissitudes of the TAT pictures has been published by W. G. Morgan (1995).

[3]Editor's note: Presumably, the "stimulating power" of these cards—the amount of information their stories contributed to the diagnosis of each participant under study at the HPC—was less than that of the cards that were kept for the final TAT, Series D (see W. Morgan, chap. 6, this volume).

Card 7.   This is a drawing of a nude man and young woman in a partial embrace. To the right is an older woman wearing a robe and holding a baby in her arms. In the upper background is what appears to be two figures huddled together; the nude man is pointing to them. Below these two figures is a single figure sitting with his or her head on his or her knees. This figure is drawn in the same shaded style as that of the older woman holding the infant.

Card 12 F.   This is a drawing of a young woman with a quizzical expression on her face. Her bent arms are raised up around her head. Other figures sketched behind and in front of the woman include a robot-like figure, a light socket, an alarm clock, a long fluorescent light bulb, and an instrument with a lever that suggests a credit card compressor.

Card 14 M.   This card shows only the upper torso of a man. The picture is of his right arm raised straight up and his mouth and eyes open wide as if he is screaming.

Card 16 F.   In an outdoor scene, three young, smiling women hold out sticks over a campfire. The women are crouched together.

Card 18.   A man with bushy black hair is wearing round glasses and a long, dark coat over a shirt and tie. His face shows a stern expression and his right hand is lifted as a clenched fist.

Card 19 F.   Two female figures wearing long dresses stand looking out of tall glass windows.

Card 19 M.   Two men stand together under an archway, with their backs to the viewer. They appear to be looking out at some trees.

Card 20.   In a drawing on a black background, white lines suggest a demonic head at the top and a second eerie-looking figure below. Other lines in the background suggest a tree, water, and lightning.

At the Western State Psychiatric Institute and the University of Pittsburgh

Pioneer Research on Norms for the TAT

Neither C. Morgan nor Murray obtained and afforded other examiners scoring norms for the TAT; neither did other psychologists who advocated the technique in the early years. In general, the method was used like a structured interview, as a tool that depends for its validity on the training and experience of the examiner. An example of such an approach is found in *The Thematic Apperception Test: An Introductory Manual for Its Clinical Use With Adults* (Stein, 1948). In this manual, considerable dependence on "intuitive" analysis is involved, even though the author recognized the dangers of such a reliance. In my original research on norms conducted at WSPI beginning in 1943, my aim was to supply standards for scoring, analysis, and interpretation of the TAT similar to those available for psychometric tests. The similarities and differences from psychometric measurement are discussed in "Apperceptive Norms for the Thematic Apperception Test" (Rosenzweig, 1949a).

Around this same time, I offered what was probably the first comprehensive course on projective methods, including the Rorschach test, TAT, and others. In connection with this instruction at the University of Pittsburgh, a seminar on the TAT was conducted in 1944–1945 and involved the collaboration of 11 students who gathered stories for selected cards from a total of 50 male and 50 female examinees (cf. Rosenzweig & Fleming, 1949). An earlier article addresses the problem of norms in psychometric vis-à-vis projective methods and makes the distinction between *apperceptive* (descriptive) and *thematic* (interpretive) norms for the TAT (Rosenzweig, 1949a). The collaborators in the seminar gathered most of the data for the apperceptive norms, which were later presented in an article by Rosenzweig and Fleming (1949). In a project that became the basis for her master's thesis, Fleming (1946) further analyzed the results obtained at a preliminary stage by the students and added data from 17 other participants. The resulting apperceptive norms, intended for clinical and research uses, were published in 1949. They were extensively presented as Table 1 under the headings Figures, Objects, Problems, and Outcomes. Other quantitative norms were presented in three additional tables.

The TAT norms were applied conscientiously in clinical work and training at WSPI while I was the chief psychologist (1943–1949) and were used in the CPM of TAT analysis described below. These norms were also used in my clinical training and teaching at Washington University in St. Louis (MO) beginning in 1949.

Composite Portrait Method of Thematic Apperception Test Analysis

While at Pittsburgh, I also devised a new method for analyzing and interpreting the TAT, namely, the CPM. This method was an adaptation of Francis Galton's "Composite Portraits" (1878) and "Generic Images" (1879), which had been separately published by him and then incorporated as chapters of his famous book *Inquiries Into Human Faculty and Its Development* (Galton, 1883). He introduced these methods in 1878 and 1879, respectively. Generic images was based on "blended memories" and, as he explained in his presentation at the Royal Institution, was conceived by an analogy with the composite portraits described a year earlier. The topic of blended memories has become very timely today when in connection with adult recall of childhood sexual and other abuse, a whole epidemic of forensic cases has permeated the public arena since approximately 1980. In that context, psychologists would do well to consult Galton's exposition, which is conveniently reprinted in *Inquiries*.

My present concern is with the adaptation of these methods, originally devised by Galton, to the TAT. My intention was to go from composite portraits and generic images to TAT analysis by considering the insights afforded by the TAT as, in essence, a creative expression of the individual who is reorganizing his or her previous experiences as retained in his or her memory. The assumption of the composite portrait procedure is that each of the pictures elicits memory images and that just as Galton combined photographic images for purposes of generalization, one can combine memory images that express the individual personality. Combined systematically by an adaptation of Galton's procedure, a generic portrait of the individual personality can be obtained. To accomplish this result, one needs, of course, to take account of the apperceptive aspects of the examinee's responses as well as the thematic aspects for each stimulus picture, which can then be applied in an attempt to understand the particular individual. As explained above, these two types of norms for selected pictures were obtained by specialized investigation.

The CPM of TAT analysis was described and illustrated in the book *Psychodiagnosis,* which I published in 1949(b) in collaboration with Kogan (see pp. 139–159). This exposition was included with similar ones for other current projective methods, such as the Word Association Test and the Rorschach method. Further details are available in the book, where the exposition is followed by two illustrative protocols.

In the CPM, it is assumed that the examinee projects himself or herself into the stories by identifying with the central characters and that the figures and themes with which the stories are populated represent the population of the particular idioverse (the population of events for a particular individual or a concept substituted for personality). The particular ways in which the examinee responds to a picture or relates the characters to each other are hypothetically assumed to be representative of the individual (see Hermans, chap. 16, this volume, regarding how a similar TAT approach can be used in narrative therapy). The recurrence of unique features from story to story provides the other main basis for interpretation.

Application of the Thematic Apperception Test to Therapy

In 1948, I published an article on the use of the TAT in diagnosis and therapy. A related publication, in collaboration with a psychiatrist at WSPI, appeared a year earlier (Rosenzweig & Isham, 1947). One section of the 1948 article deals with psychiatric diagnosis in much the same way that the Rorschach method had been used earlier. But a longer and more important section deals with "dynamic diagnosis." In this regard, the article was a preliminary discussion of the CPM as described in the book *Psychodiagnosis* (Rosenzweig, 1949b).

The major contribution of the article is the section on psychotherapy that explores the use of the TAT as a guide to therapy (Rosenzweig, 1948). Two general approaches are discussed. The first application is fairly active and direct and involves interpretations made by a therapist to a patient.

Here, the therapist derives knowledge of the patient's personality from the administered TAT and then imparts it, with or without supporting evidence, from the test data. The more nondirective approach involves interpretations made chiefly by the patient for himself or herself as a result of free associations to the stories. In this manner, the TAT may be particularly valuable in terms of inducing catharsis, in overcoming a block in therapy, and in the abreaction of grief and disappointment. Also discussed is the close relationship between the TAT approach and the method of dream analysis used by Freud in the early days of psychoanalysis. One difference, however, is that there tends to be a lesser degree of distortion in stories than in dreams, making TAT productions a readier object of analysis for brief psychotherapy. Finally, it was recognized that this short article is merely an introduction intended to stimulate research in more detail by others. A valuable part of the article is the list of references, which, for the date in question, was fairly exhaustive.

Validation of the Triadic Hypothesis

The TAT was used as one tool in the experimental validation of the triadic hypothesis, which I formulated in a contribution to Murray's *Explorations* (Rosenzweig, 1938, pp. 472–490). The triadic hypothesis is as follows: "Hypnotizability as a personality trait is to be found in positive association with repression as a preferred mechanism of defense and with impunitiveness as a characteristic type of immediate reaction to frustration" (Rosenzweig, 1938, p. 489).

As a corollary to the triadic hypothesis, nonhypnotizability could be associated with such other defense mechanisms as displacement and projection and with other types of reaction to frustration, namely, intropunitiveness and extrapunitiveness. Explicitly, this hypothesis emerged from an experimental study of repression in which it appeared that individuals who used or failed to use this mechanism of defense were differentiated also in the character of their immediate reactions to frustration. On the one hand, those who tended to forget their failures, in accordance with the repression theory, seemed to react in the frustrating situation itself by glossing over and rationalizing (impunitive). On the other hand, those who were prone to remember their failures better than their successes, and hence could not be said to have repressed their unpleasant experiences, seemed to respond in the frustrating situation with aggression directed either outwardly (extrapunitive) or inwardly (intropunitive). It was speculated that both the extrapunitive and intropunitive reactions entailed remembering the occasion of frustration as if, in the former case, in the anticipation of revenge and, in the latter, in preparation for nursing the wounds to one's pride. In either case, the aggressive impulses arising in the immediately frustrating situation tended to be preserved for later expression as, for example, in memory. By contrast, the impunitive reaction was conceived to entail a conscious forgetting of the frustrating experience as if in keeping with the motive of reconciling one's self and others to the disagreeable situation.

The data and results for the TAT were presented by Rosenzweig and Sarason (1942; see also Sarason, 1942). These results indicate the profitable application of the TAT in the investigation of theoretical constructs in the area of personality. A related project was conducted by Korchin (1943) in a comparative study of three projective techniques used for the study of the measurement of frustration-reaction types.

Further investigation led to more systematic classification of frustration-reaction types and to the development of a new projective psychodiagnostic technique, the Rosenzweig Picture-Frustration Study (Rosenzweig, 1978a, 1978b). This apperceptive method continues to be used worldwide.

Thematic Apperception as an Approach to the Study of Creativity

The application of the TAT to the study of creativity appeared as a centenary contribution to the writings of Henry James (Rosenzweig, 1943). It bears the title "The Ghost of Henry James: A Study in Thematic Apperception." This article first appeared in the psychological journal *Character & Personality* but was promptly requested for reprinting in the prestigious *Partisan Review* (Rosenzweig, 1943). As a chapter, it was also later included in three edited books. This study was followed by a contribution dealing more generally with the James family under the title "The James's Stream of Consciousness" (Rosenzweig, 1958), which traces the concept of the title from Galton's studies on word association to Freud's method of free association and the literary stream of consciousness exemplified by James, Sr. and, more explicitly and in more detail, by James, Jr. in his fictional writings. The concinnity among the father and the two brothers, William and Henry, constituted a contribution to the understanding of the creative process.

In a more recent monograph (Rosenzweig, 1987) under the title "Sally Beauchamp's Career: A Psychoarcheological Key to Morton Prince's Classic Case of Multiple Personality," I used what I called "psychoarchaeology" to reconstruct the psychological biography of a New England woman treated by Prince. This method is a modification of the TAT approach to thematic content analysis. It is closely derived from Freud's methods of dream interpretation. Prince, a colleague of William James, founded HPC in 1927, with Murray as his assistant and later his successor. The multiple personality of Sally Beauchamp—a case of great renown in the history of psychology—made Prince, who became a professor of abnormal psychology at Harvard University shortly before his death in 1929, a universally recognized authority on this baffling mental disorder. The 500-page biographical study Prince published about the case in 1906 was meant to catch the attention of the professional and public readership by its sensational revelations, yet its awkward style left even the professional reader mystified.

The origins of the disorder were never truly explained. The volume was a tour de force thrown into the teeth of the rival psychoanalytic school of Freud that championed unconscious psychodynamics. To this approach, Prince opposed the structural subconscious and "coconscious." In this perspective, he selectively presented his records of the Beauchamp treatment. But even the bare bones of the patient's biography, let alone the dynamics, were so concealed, partly to protect the privacy of the patient, that a dubious and only temporary triumph was achieved.

The remaining puzzle was at last unraveled. By the exercise of what was designated psychoarchaeological reconstruction, almost every important detail of the biography was recovered, despite the author's deliberate omissions and disguises. At a distance of nearly a century, the actual identity of the patient and other revelations became permissible. In addition, the dynamics of the case were then strikingly demonstrated. It turns out that this classic case had a remarkably modern ring. For example, the effects of child abuse, today being so widely investigated, were disclosed as relevant to this history. Evident also were the effects of sudden infant death syndrome, which has been recognized and formulated as SIDS in medical circles only within the last 15 years, with the etiology still unsolved. But a child's experience of this syndrome in the family history was clearly shown as highly pertinent to the development of personality dissociation. It is likely that its relevance in this case will prove to bear on a broad range of psychopathology.

To a certain extent the application of the TAT to the study of creativity is a tributary to the general approach to human behavior and personality, which I introduced in 1950–1951 under the name "idiodynamics." In fact, idiodynamics as such was initially presented in conjunction with the projective techniques, including the TAT (Rosenzweig, 1951, 1985). Idiodynamics focuses on the unique phenomenal world of each individual, with its several levels of expression and various modes of communication. It entails attention to explicit and implicit conscious processes and implicit unconscious processes, such as those revealed by the TAT (see Rosenzweig, 1992, 1994, for a more definitive illustration of applied idiodynamics). The TAT and idiodynamics are outgrowths of empathically informed scientific approaches to expanding psychologists' self-awareness by recognizing the creative artist in each individual.

References

Douglas, C. (1993). *Translate this darkness: The life of Christiana Morgan.* New York: Simon & Schuster.

Douglas, C. (1997). *Visions: Notes of the seminar given in 1930–1934 by C. G. Jung.* Princeton, NJ: Princeton University Press.

Fleming, E. E. (1946). *A descriptive analysis of responses in the Thematic Apperception Test.* Unpublished master's thesis, University of Pittsburgh.

Galton, F. (1878). Composite portraits. *Nature, 18,* 97–100.

Galton, F. (1879). Generic images. *Proceedings of the Royal Institution, 9,* 161–170.

Galton, F. (Ed.). (1883). *Inquiries into human faculty and its development.* London: Macmillan.

Jung, C. J. (1976). *The visions seminars.* Zurich: Spring.

Korchin, S. J. (1943). *A comparative study of three projective techniques in the measurement of frustration-reaction types.* Master's thesis, Clark University, Worcester, MA.

Morgan, C. D., & Murray, H. A. (1935). A method for investigating fantasies: The Thematic Apperception Test. *Archives of Neurology and Psychiatry, 34,* 289–306.

Morgan, W. G. (1995). Origin and history of the Thematic Apperception Test images. *Journal of Personality Assessment, 65,* 237–254.

Murray, H. A. (Ed.). (1938). *Explorations in personality: A clinical and experimental study of fifty men of college age.* New York: Oxford University Press.

Murray, H. A. (1943). *The Thematic Apperception Test: Manual.* Cambridge, MA: Harvard University Press.

Prince, M. (1906). *The dissociation of a personality: A biographical study in abnormal psychology.* New York: Longmans.

Robinson, F. G. (1992). *Love's story told: A life of Henry A. Murray.* Cambridge, MA: Harvard University Press.

Rosenzweig, S. (1938). The experimental study of repression. In H. A. Murray (Ed.), *Explorations in personality* (pp. 472–490). New York: Oxford University Press.

Rosenzweig, S. (1943). The ghost of Henry James: A study in thematic apperception. *Character & Personality, 12,* 79–100.

Rosenzweig, S. (1948). The thematic apperception technique in diagnosis and therapy. *Journal of Personality, 16,* 437–444.

Rosenzweig, S. (1949a). Apperceptive norms for the Thematic Apperception Test: The problem of norms in projective methods. *Journal of Personality, 17,* 475–482.

Rosenzweig, S. (with Kogan, K. L.). (1949b). Thematic Apperception Test. In *Psychodiagnosis* (pp. 139–159). New York: Grune & Stratton.

Rosenzweig, S. (1951). Idiodynamics in personality theory with special reference to projective methods. *Psychological Review, 58,* 213–223.

Rosenzweig, S. (1958). The James's stream of consciousness. *Contemporary Psychology, 3,* 250–257.

Rosenzweig, S. (1978a). *Aggressive behavior and the Rosenzweig Picture-Frustration Study.* New York: Praeger.

Rosenzweig, S. (1978b). *The Rosenzweig Picture-Frustration (P-F) Study: Basic manual.* St. Louis, MO: Rana House.

Rosenzweig, S. (1985). Freud and experimental psychology: The emergence of idiodynamics. In S. Koch & D. E. Leary (Eds.), *A century of psychology as science* (pp. 135–207). New York: McGraw-Hill.

Rosenzweig, S. (1987). Sally Beauchamp's career: A psychoarcheological key to Morton Prince's classic case of multiple personality. *Genetic, Social, and General Psychology Monographs, 113,* 5–60.

Rosenzweig, S. (1992). *Freud, Jung, and Hall the king-maker: The historic expedition to American (1909) with G. Stanley Hall as host and William James as guest.* Seattle, WA: Hogrefe & Huber.

Rosenzweig, S. (1994). *The historic expedition to America (1909): Freud, Jung, and Hall the king-maker with G. Stanley Hall as host and William James as guest* (2nd ed.). St. Louis, MO: Rana House.

Rosenzweig, S., & Fleming, E. E. (1949). Apperceptive norms for the Thematic Apperception Test. II: An empirical investigation. *Journal of Personality, 17,* 483–503.

Rosenzweig, S., & Isham, A. C. (1947). Complementary Thematic Apperception Test patterns in close kin. *American Journal of Orthopsychiatry, 17,* 129–142.

Rosenzweig, S., & Sarason, S. (1942). An experimental study of the triadic hypothesis: Reaction to frustration, ego-defense and hypnotizability. I: Correlational approach. *Character & Personality, 11,* 1–19.

Sarason, S. (1942). *Relationship of reaction to frustration, ego-defense, and suggestibility: An experimental study of the triadic hypothesis.* Doctoral dissertation, Clark University, Worcester, MA.

Stein, M. I. (1948). *The Thematic Apperception Test: An introductory manual for its clinical use with adults.* Cambridge, MA: Addison-Wesley.

Part III

Artistic and Literary Influences

5

Look Homeward, Harry: Literary Influence on the Development of the Thematic Apperception Test

Lon Gieser and Wesley G. Morgan

The Thematic Apperception Test (TAT) is steeped in literature. The profound literary immersion of the life and personal identity of its creator, Harry Murray, has been explicated by his biographers, Forrest Robinson (1992, and personal communication, April 4, 1995) and James W. Anderson (1988, 1990, and chap. 6, this volume). Murray, declared Robinson (1992), "was almost literally 'made' out of books" (p. 385). He was a voracious reader of novels, plays, and poetry and was well schooled in the classics; Murray even published literary criticism—the product of his passionate avocation as a Melville scholar.

During "a head-long plunge into the arts" in the early 1920s, for example, Murray bought and read "Shakespeare, the English Romantic poets, Tolstoy, Chekhov, and Dostoevsky, along with the major American writers" (Robinson, 1992, p. 92). Among the literary figures he encountered were Sherwood Anderson, F. Scott Fitzgerald, Edmund Wilson, and Eugene O'Neill. Murray was so enthralled by the Broadway stage that he "had a theatre of his own built on his farm at Topsfield, Massachusetts, where he and his friends and students performed psychodrama, using, on occasions, a variety of masks which he had constructed at the Metropolitan Opera" (Shneidman, 1981, p. 559).

The influence of literature on the TAT was acknowledged by Murray. In the article introducing the TAT, Christiana Morgan and Murray (1935/1981) noted that

> another fact which was relied on in devising the present method is that a great deal of written fiction is the conscious or unconscious expression of the author's experiences or fantasies. The process involved is that of projection—something well known to analysts. (pp. 390–391)

Participants in early TAT research were asked to "indulge their literary imagination" (Morgan & Murray, 1938, p. 532).

In this chapter, we address further literary aspects of the TAT enterprise. Drawing on the recollections of Nevitt Sanford, one of Murray's colleagues who helped develop the TAT, we reveal the likely literary influence of Thomas Wolfe's (1957) novel *Look Homeward, Angel* on the TAT's genesis.

For Murray, wonder was the grace of psychology. His wish was to explore the mysteries of the human condition and its unique personalities by binding art with science, so as to avoid psychological reductionism. Murray was lured into this expansive approach by reading Melville's *Moby-Dick* in 1924 (Murray, 1943b, 1953). Its overarching archetypal dramatization of the conflict between the unconscious forces and the conscious strivings of the human soul moved Murray to devote himself to deepening his understanding of himself and others.

Novelists like Melville have the remarkable ability to limn with enlightening empathy, a vast array of human relationships. Readers are given insight into the joys, sorrows, frustrations, consolations, blessings, and delusions they all face in their everyday lives on rational, emotional, and spiritual levels. One is provided with other perspectives of how the present is shaped and measured by the past and of how much the future of one's life is in the hands of fate.

The reader who is enchanted with literature, as Murray was, can readily experience imagery intended by the author's words. When readers become enveloped by the imagery along with the aesthetic and emotional tone of the words, they may find themselves participating in the moods, attitudes, and values underlying the author's creativity. The author's expression induces a corresponding process of reception in the reader that joins the reader to the author. Some would say that literature exists in this transformative union. Intense identification with the author's characters results in what Mellville termed the "shock of recognition," which impels the reader to experience himself and the world anew.

The beauty of literature is that it can open "a serene and luminous region of truth where all may meet and expiate in common . . . [above] . . . the smoke and stir, the din and turmoil of men's lower life of care and business and debate" (Baldick, 1983, p. 103). Reading literature is a humanizing pursuit that enriches "factual" approaches to understanding oneself and others. Fictions in the form of myths and stories may indeed surpass facts as revelations of truth.

D. H. Lawrence was correct in concluding that so much of life is lived on the trivial level. But people do not *experience* their own lives on the trivial level. Quoting John Keats, Murray (1943b) asserted that

> they are a very shallow people who take everything literally. A Man's life of any worth is continual allegory, and very few eyes can see the Mystery of his life—a life like the scriptures figurative. . . . Shakespeare led a life of Allegory: his works are the comments. (p. 142)

People all lead lives of allegory. The TAT gives them incentive to make their comments.

Incidentally, one of the most important teachings of the scriptures—whether taken literally or figuratively—is that people are created in the image of God. This means that in every human being, there is a "divine spark," making each human life sacred and of infinite worth. In consequence, a human being cannot be viewed as a mere functionary in society but must be considered a unique personality. It is therefore paramount that human personality be respected in every human being. Such respect underlies Murray's vision of the TAT.

According to novelist James Caroll (1996),

> the imagination itself is sacred. All of our greatest art, music, architecture, and poetry proclaim it as such, and so do the more modest efforts of ordinary writers. . . . For [one] imbued with this idea, the very act of story-telling, of arranging memory and invention according to the structure of narrative, is by definition holy. It is a version, however finite, of what the infinite God does. Telling our stories is what saves us; the story is enough. (p. 267)

Everybody has a core of stories—emotional memories infused with imagination—with tragic and heroic plots that they live and relive within themselves consciously and unconsciously. These stories, which are elicited by TAT fantasy, influence and reflect the relationship between oneself and one's world—the very expression of personality. The TAT dramatizes personality. It embodies the confrontation of character with circumstance and elevates each person to the stature of protagonist and creative author in portraying his or her approach to life. (This has particular value in narrative therapy, as Hermans, chap. 16, this volume, demonstrates.)

Sigmund Freud demonstrated that through fantasies, and especially dreams, people reveal deeper aspects of their personalities. Carl Jung saw fantasy as manifesting archetypal imagery of the personal and universal narratives by which people live their lives and form themselves. Murray resonated with these perspectives, advancing the primacy of human imagination.

In a charming essay entitled "The Relation of the Poet to Day-Dreaming"—undoubtedly read by Murray—Freud (1908/1959) proposed that the imaginative stories of writers may be traced not only to the writer's recent experience but also to childhood memories "stirred up" by the recent experience. The memories, according to Freud, arouse basic wishes or fundamental longings that are fulfilled in the writer's production of fantasy. Given the knowledge of the writer's life, these wishes may be discerned by the reader. With amusingly Jungian overtones, Freud (1908/1959) also recognized the role of "the racial treasure house of myths, legends and fairy-tales" (p. 182) in many imaginative works, speculating that myths are "distorted vestiges of the wish-phantasies of whole nations—the age-long dreams of young humanity" (p. 182). Freud implied that in some sense people are all poets and novelists, albeit with few possessing the inexplicable literary talent to move others.

In his autobiographical portrait, Murray (1967) revealed that

> the notion that science is the creative product of an engagement between the scientist's psyche and event to which he is attentive prepared

him for an enthusiastic embracement of Jung's *Psychological Types* on
the very day of its timely publication in New York (1923). (p. 289)

Murray and Morgan's initial friendship in 1923 was largely centered
around a shared interest in Jung's book (Douglas, 1993; Robinson, 1992).

Jung (1923/1964) wrote of the "conception of a dream or phantasy in
which the persons or conditions appearing therein are related to subjective
factors entirely belonging to the subject's own psyche" (p. 599). He observed that one's "sense-perceptions and their *apperceptions*" (emphasis
added, p. 599) in daily life are similarly "subjectively conditioned." That
is, the images (*imagos*) one forms of other people definitely differ to some
extent from their "real existence." When an imago is of an extremely subjective origin, according to Jung, it is actually more an image of the relationship between the object (the other person) and one's psyche than of
the object itself; he termed this relationship a *subjective function-complex*.
Jung (1923/1964) explicitly applied this concept to "literary works, in
which the individual figures represent relatively autonomous function-
complexes in the psyche of the poet" (p. 601).

Murray (1943b) was also careful to "distinguish between fantasy—
drifting and undirected thought—and creative imagination—that is or-
ganized and oriented toward the attainment of an exacting aesthetic standard" (p. 152). To him, TAT stories are "more analogous to works of art"
(p. 152), hence they are products of creative imagination. Such thinking
brings us to our examination of the collusion of Murray's and Wolfe's creative imaginations in devising the TAT.

Murray's Novel Idea

I (Gieser) had the good fortune of being a student of Nevitt Sanford's
(1909–1995) at the Wright Institute (Berkeley, CA) from 1977 to 1980.
The eminent ego psychologist was best known for his coauthorship of *The
Authoritarian Personality* (Adorno, Frenkel-Brunswik, Levinson, & Sanford, 1950), Sanford was a Harvard University's Department of Psychology
graduate student and faculty member with Murray at the Harvard Psychological Clinic from 1931 until 1940.

Murray, the man and his methods, was a topic of Sanford and my
discussion throughout our work on personality assessment (i.e., Gieser,
1980; Gieser & Sanford, 1980; Sanford, 1982, 1985). Our research was, of
course, in the "personological" tradition of Murray's clinic. Case studies
were conducted using a multitude of life history interviews, questionnaires, psychological inventories, and projective tests—including the TAT.

Sanford was among those who helped Murray select pictures for the
TAT, and he wrote the first manual (Sanford, 1939), which was mimeo-
graphed and privately distributed 4 years before Murray's (1943b) familiar
version was published. He also coauthored two other preliminary manuals
(White & Sanford, 1941; White, Sanford, Murray, & Bellak, 1941). The
Murray–Sanford scoring scheme was an early quantitative procedure for

analyzing TAT stories (Sanford, 1941; Sanford, Adkins, Miller, & Cobb, 1943), from which Morris Stein (1955) adapted the internal "need" and environmental "press" variables for his own TAT manual. Murray (1943b, 1951/1965) publicly expressed his gratitude for Sanford's contributions to the TAT project.

Sanford told me (Gieser) that when he took Murray's personality course in 1930 (as a Harvard student not yet affiliated with the clinic), Murray had been reading Wolfe's (1929/1957) *Look Homeward, Angel.* Murray brought the book with him to several lectures, so Sanford knew that Murray was very familiar with it. "About the same time," according to Sanford (1978/1980), "[Murray] produced the early version of a projective test based on a set of evocative but ambiguous drawings, a 'thematic apperception test,' or what was intended to be one" (p. 111).

When Sanford took the time to read *Look Homeward, Angel,* he discovered that the protagonist, Eugene Gant, at school in a fictional Southern town, Altamount—a thinly veiled version of Wolfe's hometown, Asheville, North Carolina—is asked along with other children to write about a picture they had been shown. Eugene wrote a story that revealed much of his personality and potential not exhibited by his other behaviors. Sanford was persuaded that the TAT was inspired, or at least prenatally influenced, by this incident of Wolfe's. Read the passage in *Look Homeward, Angel* for yourself:

> He [the principal] had called the school together that day to command it to write him a composition. The children sat, staring dumbly up at him as he made a rambling explanation of what he wanted. Finally he announced a prize. He would give five dollars from his own pocket to the student who wrote the best paper. That aroused them. There was a rustle of interest.
>
> They were to write a paper on the meaning of a French picture called *The Song of the Lark.* It represented a French peasant girl, barefooted, with a sickle in one hand, and with face upturned in the morning-light of the fields as she listened to the bird-song. They were asked to describe what there was in the expression of the girl's face. They were asked to tell what the picture meant to them. It had been reproduced in one of their readers. A larger print was now hung up on the platform for their inspection. (Wolfe, 1929/1957, p. 172)[1]

The Song of the Lark (Le Chant de l'Alouette) was painted by Jules (Adolphe Aimé Louis) Breton in Couriérs, France, in the fall of 1884 (see Maxon, 1970; and Sturges, 1982). It depicts a young peasant girl, Marie Bédoul, barefoot at sunrise on her way to work in the fields with a sickle in her hand pausing to listen to a birdsong. Wolfe probably became acquainted with the once-popular painting, which has been on exhibit in Chicago since 1893, through his familiarity with the works of Willa Cather. In 1901, Cather first wrote of the painting in a newspaper article:

---

[1]From *Look Homeward, Angel,* by T. Wolfe, 1929, New York: Scribner, a Division of Simon & Schuster. Copyright 1929 by Charles Scribner's Sons; copyright renewed © 1957 by Edward C. Ashwell, Administrator, C.T.A. and/or Fred Wolfe. Reprinted with permission.

> You will find hundreds of merchants and farmer boys all over Nebraska and Kansas and Iowa who remember Jules Breton's beautiful "Song of the Lark," and perhaps the ugly little peasant girl standing barefooted among the wheat fields in the early morning has taught some of these people to hear the lark sing for themselves. (Curtin, 1970, pp. 842–843)

Cather (1915/1943) later wrote a semiautobiographical novel with the same title in which the painting plays an important symbolic role in awakening the protagonist's sensitivity to beauty. A reproduction of the painting (in partial silhouette) even appeared on the novel's first edition dust jacket (Rosowski, 1987; Woodress, 1987). As stated previously, Wolfe was quite familiar with Cather's work and specifically mentioned *The Song of the Lark* in one of his notebooks; in another place, Wolfe ranked Cather as the third best woman writer (Kennedy & Reeves, 1970).

Wolfe (1929/1957) continued the description of the assignment with the following:

> Sheets of yellow paper were given them. They stared, thoughtfully masticating their pencils. Finally, the room was silent save for a minute scratching on paper.
>
> The warm wind spouted about the eaves; the grasses bent, whistling gently.
>
> Eugene wrote: "The girl is hearing the song of the first lark. She knows that it means Spring has come. She is about seventeen or eighteen years old. Her people are very poor, she has never been anywhere. In the winter she wears wooden shoes. She is making out as if she was going to whistle. But she doesn't let on to the bird that she has heard him. The rest of her people are behind her, coming down the field, but we do not see them.
>
> She has a father, a mother, and two brothers. They have worked hard all their life. The girl is the youngest child. She thinks she would like to go away somewhere and see the world. Sometimes she hears the whistle of a train that is going to Paris. She has never ridden on a train in her life. She would like to go to Paris. She would like to have some fine clothes, she would like to travel. Perhaps she would like to start life new in America, the Land of Opportunity.
>
> The girl has had a hard time. Her people do not understand her. If they saw her listening to the lark they would poke fun at her. She had never had the advantages of a good education, her people are so poor, but she would profit by her opportunity if she did, more than some people who have. You can tell by looking at her that she's intelligent." (pp. 172–173)[2]

Needless to say, the 11-year-old Southern country boy Eugene won the contest. Furthermore, he was recruited to the private school begun by the principal and his wife. "That was what the paper had been for," wrote Wolfe (1929/1957, p. 208).

---

[2]From *Look Homeward, Angel,* by T. Wolfe, 1929, New York: Scribner, a Division of Simon & Schuster. Copyright 1929 by Charles Scribner's Sons; copyright renewed © 1957 by Edward C. Ashwell, Administrator, C.T.A. and/or Fred Wolfe. Reprinted with permission.

This fictional episode, it turns out, was based on a real event in Wolfe's own life (Donald, 1987; Turnbull, 1967; Wheaton, 1961). In 1912, when Wolfe was 11 years old, he was selected for a private school by virtue of his performance on a writing task in which all the boys in the sixth grade were read a story and told to reproduce it in their own words—but there was no picture.

Wolfe thus devised the visual stimulus and the TAT-like storytelling procedure for his fictional version. He used them as a vehicle to give the reader psychological insight into Eugene's makeup that would not have otherwise occurred if he had merely recounted what actually happened to him. There are other examples in literature and film where the picture-story technique is used. Following a tip from David Winter, an anachronistic, fictional version of Murray's TAT was found in the novel *Compulsion* (Levin, 1956), which dramatizes the 1924 Leopold and Loeb murder trial. In a juvenile work (Wells, 1959), a nurse observed a psychiatrist administering a fictional TAT. Another fictional TAT appeared in the comedy *The Scout* (Twentieth Century Fox, 1994), where a psychiatrist evaluates an emotionally unstable pitching prospect for the New York Yankees.

In *Explorations in Personality,* Morgan and Murray (1938) noted that TAT participants were originally instructed

> to interpret the action in each picture and make a plausible guess as to the preceding event, and the final outcome. . . . Only by experience did we discover that much more personality is revealed if the [participant] is asked to create a dramatic fiction rather than to guess at probable facts. (p. 531)

It is interesting to note that Eugene was not asked to make up a story but simply to write a composition on the meaning of the picture—instructions similar to those first tried by Murray. This may indeed be a case of life imitating art.

A Literary Psychologist

Sanford told me (Gieser) that Murray considered the study of literature to be part of psychology. Soon after Murray returned to Harvard as a research fellow, he recommended a list of books to read in modern psychology. Besides the likely works by Freud, Jung, Pierre Janet, William James, and so forth, he also recommended volumes of "psychological biography" by Katherine Anthony, Joseph Wood Krutch, and Van Wyck Brooks (Murray, 1927), probably referring to *Catherine the Great* (Anthony, 1925), *Edgar Allen Poe* (Krutch, 1926), *John Addington Symonds: A Biography* (Brooks, 1914), and *The Pilgrimage of Henry James* (Brooks, 1925). His students were expected to read biographies and novels, with which the clinic's library became well stocked after he was made director. In the spring of 1929, as a young graduate student, B. F. Skinner took one of Murray's courses, "The Psychology of the Individual." The assigned text was a biography that had been used by Gordon Allport (1929) in his personality course at Princeton University, namely, *The Locomotive God,* by the phobic poet–professor, William Ellery Leonard (1927). After the first lecture, Skinner accused Murray of being a *"literary psychologist"* (Skinner, 1979). No wonder the TAT was partly created from a fictional account of a method for evoking fantasies that appeared in an autobiographical novel.

Saul Rosenzweig and Robert White both also recalled discussions of Wolfe's works at the clinic. Lewis Mumford, a close friend of Murray's, complained that Murray was "swept away with" Wolfe's overwritten, overdramatic works focusing on Wolfe's "general theme for life" (Robinson, 1992, p. 288). In August 1935, Murray encountered Wolfe in a Southern Pacific Railroad car headed for California. The incident was recalled by Murray in an interview with one of Wolfe's biographers: According to David Herbert Donald (1987), "[Murray] spotted Wolfe because he so greatly resembled Eugene Gant and introduced himself as a great admirer of Wolfe's novels" (p. 338). Donald also recorded Murray's comical description of Wolfe's manic mouthfuls of words and food.

The fictional Eugene makes an appearance in *Explorations in Personality* (Wolf & Murray, 1938), where a lengthy excerpt from *Look Homeward, Angel* was provided to illustrate Murray's concept of *level of aspiration,* a high level of which is exhibited in fantasy through imagined achievement. Eugene fantasizes fulfilling several heroic roles, such as football star, flying ace, Jesus Christ, and Lord Byron, in an emotionally charged manner that captured Murray's attention.

The closest link one can find is a chapter by Murray (1943a) entitled "Personality and Creative Imagination." Here, Murray drew the parallel between TAT stories and literary masterpieces by demonstrating how authors are reflected in their productions. The two main authors, given as examples, are Melville and none other than Wolfe.

Murray informed readers of his vast knowledge of Wolfe's series of autobiographical novels. He included mention of a trip to Asheville, North Carolina, during which he went so far (or dove so deep) as to visit Wolfe's mother, whom he found uncannily similar to the mother portrayed in Wolfe's novels. Of his conversation with Wolfe's mother, Murray (1943a) stated, "she entertained me with an unsparing tide of talk about [her] family, which checked with what every [Wolfe] reader knows" (p. 151). A mention of meeting Wolfe on the train was also made, and Murray (1943a) told of being "at the receiving end of a torrent of eloquent autobiographical phrases of which I was surprised to see in print a few months later when *The Story of a Novel* [Wolfe, 1936] was published" (p. 151).

Among Murray's (1943a) conclusions are (a) "that certain complexes predispose an individual to creative literature, and the predominant ones determine to some extent the kinds of characters, plots, and situations that will appeal to him as worthy subjects" (pp. 153–154); and (b) "these findings are confirmed by [an] examination of the works of both Melville and of Wolfe" (p. 154). He then cited the example of how "in the poetic prelude to *Look Homeward, Angel,* the symbolism of the birth trauma—

expulsion, separation from mother—is consciously adapted as the leit-motif of the entire novel" (p. 155). A reference is made to "the archetypal Pilgrimage, or Odyssey thema, a very ancient story form which appealed as much to Thomas Wolfe as it did to Melville" (p. 155).

Murray's (1949/1981) introduction to Melville's (1949) autobiographi-cal novel, *Pierre, or the Ambiguities,* again makes reference to the odyssey of Wolfe. He quoted the phrase "look homeward, angel" when discussing an autobiographical author's "aim, mostly unconscious, . . . to be reborn, to reenter and then shed the parents' cultural husk, and to grow a new conception" (p. 427).

Although not particularly pertinent to the case at hand, we cannot resist mentioning another Murray–Wolfe connection. In 1926, Murray se-cretly rented an apartment in Cambridge (MA) near Harvard Yard. "As it happened," according to Robinson (1992), "the apartment had been home a few years earlier to Kenneth Raisbek, a friend of Thomas Wolfe, who described the place in his novel, *Of Time and the River* [1935]" (p. 163). Murray discovered that like Eugene in the novel, Wolfe had visited the apartment just after his arrival at Harvard for graduate study in 1920. This apartment later served as a rendezvous for Murray and Morgan over many years of their extramarital relationship (Douglas, 1993; Robinson, 1992).

Shortly before his death, Sanford stood by his story, even though he was aware that Murray never wrote of Wolfe's TAT contribution in any publication (Sanford, personal communications, April 8, 1995, and May 6, 1995). Sanford was also certain that nothing relevant would turn up in the Murray archives at Harvard. He became uncharacteristically indig-nant when informed that one of his old cronies recommended checking there to verify his account.

There is a precedent for Murray's omitting sources of influence in his publications. For example, Murray (1938) is identified with the field of personology, which he defined as "the branch of psychology, which primar-ily concerns itself with the study of human lives and the factors that in-fluence their course, and which investigates individual differences and types of personality" (p. 4). One even finds in Murray's obituary in *The New York Times* the following: "Dr. Murray was a wordsmith of some ac-complishment and was fond of creating new words. He first used the word 'personology' to describe the study of personality" (Fowler, 1988, p. D17). However, in a footnote, Rosenzweig (1985) informed readers that "the term personology was not coined by Murray" (p. 190).

According to Rosenzweig (1985), Murray

> adopted it from a book by J. C. Smuts (1926), who introduced the term and defined it and discussed it as the science of personality as a whole. The book by Smuts greatly impressed Murray in the early 1930's [when Rosenzweig was at the Harvard Psychological Clinic], but Murray does not cite that author (p. 190).

Conclusion

Given Murray's immersion in the life and writing of Wolfe and Sanford's observation of the proximity between the time Murray was reading *Look Homeward, Angel* and the beginning of his TAT work, it is concluded that *Look Homeward, Angel,* with its TAT-like episode, was a significant influence on the genesis of the TAT, which Murray, nevertheless, chose not to publicize.

The question remains as to why Murray never formally made information concerning Wolfe's apparent role in the development of the TAT available to the psychological or literary community. Sanford (personal communication, April 8, 1995) did not have an answer and such speculation is quite beyond us. We can only turn to Murray's observation that "every man knows something about himself which he's willing to tell, he knows something about himself that he's not willing to tell; and there's something about himself that he doesn't know and can't tell" (Robinson, 1992, p. 176).

References

Adorno, T. W., Frenkel-Brunswik, E., Levinson, D. J., & Sanford, N. (1950). *The authoritarian personality.* New York: Harper & Row.

Allport, G. W. (1929). The study of personality by the intuitive method: An experiment in teaching from *The locomotive god. Journal of Abnormal and Social Psychology, 24,* 14–27.

Anderson, J. W. (1988). Henry Murray's early career: A psychobiographical exploration. *Journal of Personality, 56,* 139–171.

Anderson, J. W. (1990). The life of Henry A. Murray: 1893–1988. In A. I. Rabin, R. A. Zucker, R. A. Emmons, & S. Frank (Eds.), *Studying persons and lives* (pp. 304–383). New York: Springer.

Anthony, K. (1925). *Catherine the great.* Garden City, NY: Garden City.

Baldick, C. (1983). *The social mission of English studies.* New York: Oxford University Press.

Brooks, V. W. (1914). *John Addington Symonds: A biography.* New York: Kennerly.

Brooks, V. W. (1925). *The pilgrimage of Henry James.* New York: Dutton.

Caroll, J. (1996). *An American requiem: God, my father, and the war that came between us.* Boston: Houghton Mifflin.

Cather, W. (1943). *The song of the lark.* Boston: Houghton Mifflin. (Original work published 1915)

Curtin, W. M. (1970). Guest editor of the *Courier.* In W. M. Curtin (Ed.), *The world of the parish. Vol. 2: Willa Cather's articles and reviews, 1893–1902* (pp. 836–862). Lincoln: University of Nebraska Press.

Donald, D. H. (1987). *Look homeward: A life of Thomas Wolfe.* Boston: Little, Brown.

Douglas, C. (1993). *Translate this darkness: The life of Christiana Morgan.* New York: Simon & Schuster.

Fowler, G. (1988, June 24). Henry A. Murray is dead at 95; developer of personality theory. *The New York Times, 137,* p. D17.

Freud, S. (1959). The relation of the poet to day-dreaming. In J. Riviere (Trans. & Ed.), *Sigmund Freud: Collected papers* (Vol. 4, pp. 173–183). New York: Basic Books. (Original work published 1908)

Gieser, M. T. (1980). *"The authoritarian personality" revisited.* Unpublished doctoral dissertation, Wright Institute, Berkeley, CA.

Gieser, M. T., & Sanford, N. (1980, May). *The development of a revised E(thnocentrism) scale.* Paper presented at the meeting of the Western Psychological Association, Honolulu, HI.

Jung, C. G. (1964). *Psychological types or the psychology of individualism.* London: Routledge & Kegan Paul. (Original work published 1923)

Kennedy, R. S., & Reeves, P. (Eds.). (1970). *The notebooks of Thomas Wolfe.* Boston: Little, Brown.

Krutch, J. W. (1926). *Edgar Allen Poe.* New York: Knopf.

Leonard, W. E. (1927). *The locomotive god.* New York: Century.

Levin, M. (1956). *Compulsion.* New York: Simon & Schuster.

Maxon, J. (1970). *The Art Institute of Chicago.* New York: Harry N. Abrams.

Melville, H. (1949). *Pierre, or the ambiguities.* New York: Hendricks House.

Morgan, C. D., & Murray, H. A. (1938). Thematic Apperception Test. In H. A. Murray (Ed.), *Explorations in personality: A clinical and experimental study of fifty men of college age* (pp. 530–545). New York: Oxford University Press.

Morgan, C. D., & Murray, H. A. (1981). A method for investigation of fantasies: The Thematic Apperception Test. In E. S. Shneidman (Ed.), *Endeavors in psychology: Selections from the personology of Henry A. Murray* (pp. 390–401). New York: Harper & Row. (Original work published 1935)

Murray, H. A. (1927, January 29). What to read in psychology? *The Independent, 118,* 134–135.

Murray, H. A. (1938). Introduction. In H. A. Murray (Ed.), *Explorations in personality: A clinical and experimental study of fifty men of college age* (pp. 3–35). New York: Oxford University Press.

Murray, H. A. (1943a). Personality and creative imagination. In R. Kirk (Ed.), *English Institute annual—1942* (pp. 139–162). New York: Columbia University Press.

Murray, H. A. (1943b). *The Thematic Apperception Test: Manual.* Cambridge, MA: Harvard University Press.

Murray, H. A. (1953). In nomine diaboli. In J. Hillway & L. S. Mansfield (Eds.), *Moby-Dick centennial essays* (pp. 3–23). Dallas, TX: Southern Methodist University Press.

Murray, H. A. (1965). Uses of the Thematic Apperception Test. In B. I. Murstein (Ed.), *Handbook of projective techniques* (pp. 425–432). New York: Wiley. (Original work published 1951)

Murray, H. A. (1967). Henry A. Murray. In E. G. Boring & G. Lindzey (Eds.), *A history of psychology in autobiography* (Vol. 5, pp. 285–310). New York: Appleton-Century-Crofts.

Murray, H. A. (1981). Introduction to "Pierre." In E. E. Shneidman (Ed.), *Endeavors in psychology: Selections from the personology of Henry A. Murray* (pp. 413–481). New York: Harper & Row. (Original work published 1949)

Robinson, F. G. (1992). *Love's story told: A life of Henry A. Murray.* Cambridge, MA: Harvard University Press.

Rosenzweig, S. (1985). Freud and experimental psychology. The emergence of idiodynamics. In S. Koch & D. E. Leary (Eds.), *A century of psychology as science* (pp. 135–207). New York: McGraw-Hill.

Rosowski, S. J. (1987). Willa Cather and the French rural tradition of Breton and Millet: O pioneers! The song of the lark, and my Antonia. In H. Sturges (Ed.), *The rural vision: France and America in the late nineteenth century* (pp. 53–62). Omaha, NE: Joslyn Art Museum.

Sanford, N. (1939). *Thematic Apperception Test: Directions for administration and scoring* [Mimeograph]. Cambridge, MA: Harvard University, Harvard Psychological Clinic.

Sanford, N. (1941). Some quantitative results from the analysis of children's stories. *Psychological Bulletin, 38,* 749.

Sanford, N. (1980). Murray's clinic as a place to learn. In N. Sanford (Ed.), *Learning after college* (pp. 104–114). Orinda, CA: Montaigne. (Original work published 1978)

Sanford, N. (1982). Social psychology: Its place in personology. *American Psychologist, 37,* 896–903.

Sanford, N. (1985). What have we learned about personality? In S. Koch & D. E. Leary (Eds.), *A century of psychology as science* (pp. 490–514). New York: McGraw-Hill.

Sanford, N., Adkins, M., Miller, D., & Cobb, E. (1943). Physique, personality and scholarship [Entire issue]. *Monographs of the Society for Research in Child Development, 8*(1).

Shneidman, E. S. (1981). Introduction to Part VI: Personology encompasses a wide range of concerns, from special practical issues to human values and urgent global problems. In E. E. Shneidman (Ed.), *Endeavors in psychology: Selections from the personology of Henry A. Murray* (pp. 557–562). New York: Harper & Row.

Skinner, B. F. (1979). *The shaping of a behaviorist: Part two of an autobiography.* New York: Knopf.

Smuts, J. C. (1926). *Holism and evolution.* New York: Macmillan.

Stein, M. I. (1955). *The Thematic Apperception Test: An introductory manual for its clinical use with adults* (rev. ed.). Cambridge, MA: Addison-Wesley.

Sturges, H. (1982). Romantic evocations: Salon paintings 1880–1894. In H. Sturges (Ed.), *Jules Breton and the French rural tradition* (pp. 95–96). Omaha, NE: Joslyn Art Museum.

Turnbull, A. (1967). *Thomas Wolfe.* New York: Scribner.

Twentieth Century Fox. (1994). *The scout.* (Available from Fox Video)

Wells, H. (1959). *Cherry Ames at Hilton Hospital.* New York: Grosset & Dunlap.

Wheaton, M. W. (1961). *Thomas Wolfe and his family.* Garden City, NJ: Doubleday.

White, R. W., & Sanford, N. (1941). *Morgan–Murray Thematic Apperception Test: Manual of directions* [Mimeograph]. Cambridge, MA: Harvard University, Harvard Psychological Clinic.

White, R. W., Sanford, N., Murray, H. A., & Bellak, L. (1941). *Morgan–Murray Thematic Apperception Test: Manual of directions* [Mimeograph]. Cambridge, MA: Harvard University, Harvard Psychological Clinic.

Wolf, R., & Murray, H. A. (1938). Judgments of personality. In H. A. Murray (Ed.), *Explorations in personality: A clinical and experimental study of fifty men of college age* (pp. 243–281). New York: Oxford University Press.

Wolfe, T. (1935). *Of time and the river: A legend of man's hunger and his youth.* New York: Scribner.

Wolfe, T. (1936). *The story of a novel.* New York: Scribner.

Wolfe, T. (1957). *Look homeward, angel.* New York: Scribner. (Original work published 1929)

Woodress, J. (1987). *Willa Cather: A literary life.* Lincoln: University of Nebraska Press.

6

The 1943 Images:
Their Origin and History

Wesley G. Morgan

In this chapter, I examine each of the Thematic Apperception Test (TAT) pictures from the 1943/1971 edition of the TAT. This is the third revision of the test that was first distributed by the Harvard Psychological Clinic in 1936. This edition is printed by the Harvard University Press and the one in common use today. It is also referred to as "Series D" by Henry Murray to differentiate it from earlier editions or revisions of the test (Holt, 1946; Rapaport, Gill, & Schafer, 1946). Series A, B, and C cards were made by gluing photographs onto cardboard stock. Series D was the first series to actually have the pictures printed on cardboard stock, probably in anticipation of widespread use. Descriptions of the Series A cards can be found in "Thematic Apperception Test" (Morgan, 1938), "A Method for Investigating Fantasies" (Morgan & Murray, 1935), and "Thematic Apperception Test" (Morgan & Murray, 1938); descriptions of Series B cards can be found in *Morgan–Murray Thematic Apperception Test* (White, Sanford, Murray, & Bellak, 1941); and descriptions of the Series C cards can be found in "A Method of Administering and Evaluating the Thematic Apperception Test in Group Situations" (Clark, 1944). Work concerning the earlier editions of the TAT and the history and development of TAT images subsequent to Series D, including the TAT-II, is in progress.

Many of the pictures in Series D were suggested by members of the clinic staff other than Christiana Morgan and Murray. Murray (1943/1971) listed the specific pictures suggested by Nevitt Sanford, Frederick Wyatt, and Jurgan Ruesch in addition to Morgan. Murray (1943/1971) also mentioned "[David] Rapaport, Sanford, [David] Shakow, and others" (p. 4) in helping him with the selection of the pictures for Series D. In addition to those previously mentioned, Murray (1965) later credited Robert White, Sylvan Tomkins, Leopold Bellak, William Henry, Morris Stein, and Saul Rosenzweig in addition to Morgan as helping to shape the character of the

I thank Caroline (Nina) Murray for permission to examine the Henry A. Murray papers in the Harvard University Archives. I also thank Robert Holt, Morris Stein, and Saul Rosenzweig for their comments on earlier versions of this chapter and Lon Gieser for his editorial assistance. This chapter is a revised version with additional material of "Origin and History of the Thematic Apperception Test Images," by W. G. Morgan, 1995, *Journal of Personality Assessment, 65,* 237–252. Copyright 1995 by Erlbaum. Adapted with permission.

TAT. Thus, it would appear as if Morgan's central role in the identification of usable pictures had been diluted over time.

Several of the previous images were redrawn for Series D by the artist Samuel Thal (1903–1964). Why his services were employed rather than continuing to use the talents of Morgan remains to be explained, but again Morgan's relative artistic contribution to the Series D revision seems to have been diminished.

During the period of development of Series D, Morgan suffered from a serious health condition. She had a long-standing problem of very high blood pressure and eventually underwent a radical sympathectomy in an attempt to correct the problem. The surgery was in the fall of 1943, about the time of the publication of Series D (see Rosenzweig, chap. 4, this volume).

Murray (1943/1971) chose the cards to be used in Series D in the following manner. An unspecified number of participants ranging in age from 14 to 40 years were studied over a "considerable period" of time at the Harvard Psychological Clinic using a variety of assessment methods. The end result was a final psychological diagnosis for each participant. Each TAT story told about how each card was examined, and a rating was given to each card corresponding to the amount of information it contributed to the final diagnosis of each participant. The average of the ratings given to each card thus reflected its "stimulating power." Presumably, the cards with the greatest stimulating power were selected.

The origin and history of the current TAT cards are of interest for several reasons. First, although Murray (1943/1971) should be an unimpeachable source of such information, unfortunately the information in the *Thematic Apperception Test: Manual* is dated, often incomplete, or inaccurate. In this chapter, I attempt to correct these deficits and more completely document the original sources of the stimulus material. Second, there is the assumption that the stimuli used in projective tests contribute in an usually undefined way to the precepts reported. As Murstein (1972) maintained,

> unless we have some concept of what is there in the picture, it is difficult to decide to what degree S [the participant] is projecting personally motivated data and to what degree he is responding in a normative fashion to objectively present stimuli. (p. 145)

Although this led Holt (1978), Murstein (1972), Rosenzweig and Fleming (1949), and others to develop response norms for various groups, it has led me to a more detailed examination of the images themselves. Finally, many of the images were created for reasons other than for use in projective testing. Often the artist was attempting to communicate a thought or feeling to the observer. To the extent that this purpose is known, it is likely to be an aid in interpretation.

Thematic Apperception Test Cards

For the information that follows, Murray (1943/1971) provided the descriptions and card numbers. These are often used to identify the cards and are repeated here because of their familiarity. Cards designated with an *M* were for males (men and boys older than 14 years), with an *F* for females (women and girls older than 14 years), with a *B* for younger boys, and with a *G* for younger girls. Cards without a letter suffix were thought to be appropriate for all ages and both sexes.

I have made an attempt to identify the ultimate source of each of the images as well as reproductions of the image published before 1943 that could have served as the proximal source or inspiration for the actual TAT picture. In many cases, this identification was easy and straightforward; in other cases, the proximal image may have appeared in multiple earlier sources. There is of course no guarantee that this listing is exhaustive. Note as well that although all the TAT cards are only printed in black and white, many of the original images were created in color either as magazine illustrations or paintings. The color illustrations can be seen in the magazines where they were printed. Color reproductions of the paintings can usually be obtained from the museum where the artwork is located. Alternative sources of color reproductions are also provided where known.

Card 1

"A young boy is contemplating a violin that rests on a table in front of him." This image is one of the "old standbys." It had previously been used in Series A, Series B, and Series C. Murray (1943/1971) informed his reader that the image is a "drawing by Christina D. Morgan" (p. 18). Although this is most likely true as far as it goes, the citation by Murray does not tell the whole story. The drawing is actually a close copy of a photograph of the young violinist Yehudi Menuhin (1916–1999). A reproduction of the photograph attributed to S. Lumiere can be found in the January 1930 issue of *Parent's Magazine* and more recently in *The Music of Man* (Y. Menuhin & Davis, 1979) and *The Menuhin Saga* (M. Menuhin, 1984). Y. Menuhin maintained that the photograph was taken when he was 6 years old, the year before he made his debut with the San Francisco Symphony (Y. Menuhin & Davis, 1979), but there is some reason to doubt his account of his age. A more complete discussion of this photograph appears in "A True TAT Story" (Jahnke & Morgan, 1997).

Card 2

"Country scene: in the foreground is a young woman with books in her hand, in the background a man is working in the fields and an older woman is looking on." Murray (1943/1971) credited this picture as a "mural by Leon Kroll, reproduced by special permission of the U.S. Department of Justice" (p. 18). In fact, the American artist Leon Kroll (1884–-

1974), best known for his murals and paintings of female nudes, was commissioned to paint two lunettes for the Department of Justice.

Murray, however, misattributed the source of Card 2. The actual source of the image is a painting entitled *Morning on the Cape* done by Kroll in 1935 and now in the Museum of Art, Carnegie Institute, Pittsburgh, Pennsylvania. The painting by Kroll is evidently known by several names. Boswell (1937) referred to the title as *Fertility,* as did Holt (1978); this title seems to capture the feeling of the growth potential of the mind, land, and body so clearly illustrated in the painting. Earlier, however, Ryder (1936) referred to it as *Morning on the Cape,* and it has been called by that name by most writers after that time. Black and white reproductions of the painting can be found in "Patrons Art Fund Purchase" (O'Conner, 1935), "Carnegie Institute Acquires" (1936), "America's International Awards" (Ryder, 1936), "Leon Kroll" (Lane, 1937), and *American Painting Today* (Watson, 1939). I have been unable to find a published color reproduction of the painting. The cape referred to in the title is Cape Ann, Massachusetts.

One contemporary art writer described *Morning on the Cape* as a Spring morning with an expectant mother and a 15-year-old maiden going off to school ("Carnegie Institute Acquires," 1936). If one looks closely at the card, Kroll's signature is visible at the bottom right-hand corner. This painting was suggested for use by Ruesch and was first used in Series C. The canvas was voted "most popular" when it was shown at the Carnegie Institute International Exhibition in 1935 (Lane, 1937; O'Conner, 1935).

Card 3 BM

"On the floor against a couch is the huddled form of a boy with his head bowed on his right arm. Beside him on the floor is a revolver." Murray (1943/1971) stated that this picture, the second of the old standbys, is a drawing by Morgan. A reproduction appears in "Thematic Apperception Test" (Morgan & Murray, 1938). The card previously appeared in Series A, Series B, and Series C. The earlier pictures appear to be slightly sharper and better defined.

Actually, this drawing too comes from a photograph and is not an original composition, as Murray implied. The photograph may be found, framed along with Morgan's drawing, in the lobby of the Murray Research Center (Radcliffe College, 10 Garden St., Cambridge, MA). The photograph shows significantly more detail than the drawing, including printed material on the couch instead of a solid color, a pillow to the figure's right, and another room to the figure's left. The figure in the photograph is not wearing a belt.

Card 3 GF

"A young woman is standing with downcast head, her face covered with her right hand. Her left arm is stretched forward against a wooden door."

This picture is a black and white illustration drawn by Harold von Schmidt (1893–1982) to accompany the fourth of five installments of the serialized version of the novel, *Golden Apples* by Marjorie Kinnan Rawlings (1896–1953; Rawlings, 1935a). The illustration has the caption, "Allie had been happy that evening. It had seemed so good to have Tordell back home. But now, stumbling blindly from his room, she sobbed convulsively, knowing he no longer loved her" (Rawlings, 1935b, p. 83). The TAT picture crops off the left third and the bottom quarter of the 2-page black and white illustration.

The picture depicts young Allie Brinley, a squatter who has been living at an abandoned Florida cabin with her brother, Luke. She has fallen in love with the landowner, Richard Tordell, a recently arrived Englishman, and has become pregnant by him. Returning home after a beating by the townspeople and a talk with Luke in his room, Tordell has agreed to marry Allie. However,

> there was no quieting her. She stood a little apart, her breath convulsive. She turned and walked out the room blindly, understanding her exile. Her sobs sounded down the breezeway. They came muffled from beyond the walls of the house. They passed from hearing. (Rawlings, 1935b, p. 84)

The same image appears in Series B and Series C; Thal redrew the picture for Series D. The earlier cards show the woman with her left arm against what seems to be a paneled wall, with her right arm in a slightly different position. The Series D picture shows her left arm stretched forward against a wooden door. The description of the picture in the 1943 manual was changed to reflect the redrawing (Murray, 1943/1971).

Card 4

"A woman is clutching the shoulders of a man whose face and body are averted as if he were trying to pull away from her." This picture comes from a color illustration by an American artist and illustrator, Cecil Calvert Beall (1892–1967). It was drawn in poster style, with bold patterns of light and shadow to illustrate the short story "Best Man's Gift" by Henry Mead Williams and appeared in *Collier's* (Williams, 1940). The characters shown are Orrin Abbott, a 25-year-old lobster fisherman and partner of Grant Foster (not pictured), and Anza Cole, the recent wife of Grant Foster. The picture illustrates a scene at Orinn's fishing shack in which Anza is asking Orrin what he is going to do the following Winter. Orrin, trying to shake off feelings of attraction for Anza, says he does not know.

In the original color illustration, the woman sitting on the couch in the background with her skirt pulled up is more clearly seen as a pinup on the wall rather than, perhaps, a woman in the next room. This illustration was suggested for use by Wyatt and was first used as Card 11 in Series C.

Card 5

"A middle-aged woman is standing on the threshold of a half-opened door looking into a room." This picture comes from an illustration spread over 2 pages by W. Smithson Broadhead, drawn to accompany the first installment of an abridged and serialized novel, *The Stars Look Down* by Archibald Joseph Cronin (1896–1981; Cronin, 1935a). The illustration has the caption, " 'Hetty,' Richard Barras said quickly, 'you know I'm fond of you. I can give you—' And just at the moment Aunt Carrie opened the door" (Cronin, 1935b, p. 67). The TAT picture crops off the right side of the illustration, which shows Hetty sitting on the lap of Richard Barras while seeming to push him away. The TAT picture shows only Aunt Carrie looking into the room.

Richard Barras is a 59-year-old, wealthy owner of the Neptune Coal Mine. After a disastrous flood at the mine, he has been paying increasing attention to coquettish Hetty Todd, the recent fiancée of his son, Arthur. Aunt Caroline (Carrie) Wandless lives with the family, caring for her invalid sister, Richard's wife. Richard has recently become less inhibited in his behavior and has been giving Hetty expensive gifts. Hetty has just changed the phonograph record to a "terribly smart and catchy" dance tune and passed by the settee where Richard was sitting. Richard grabbed her by the wrist and pulled her down onto his knees. This spontaneous behavior rather surprised both of them, and Hetty simply stared at him offering no struggle. At this moment, Aunt Carrie enters the room and is shocked by the spectacle on the settee, so shocked and upset that later that evening she accidentally poisons her sister by giving her medication from the wrong bottle.

This image was first used in Series B, but it was not used in Series C. Thal redrew the image for Series D, and he seems to have made the woman appear somewhat younger and changed the style of her blouse. He also added a bookcase on the wall and books on the cabinet. The description of the picture in the 1943 manual is also changed from an "elderly" to "middle-aged" woman (Murray, 1943/1971).

Card 6 BM

"A short elderly woman stands with her back turned to a tall young man. The latter is looking downward with a perplexed expression." This drawing, another of the old standbys, was done by Morgan and used in Series A, Series B, and Series C. In the earlier cards, there was no window shown to the left of the woman. A reproduction of this earlier card appears in "Thematic Apperception Test" (Morgan & Murray, 1938).

Card 6 GF

"A young woman sitting on the edge of a sofa looks back over her shoulder at an older man with a pipe in his mouth who seems to be addressing her." This picture is taken from a black and white illustration by the American illustrator Hy Rubin (1905–1960). It was drawn to illustrate the serialized version of a mystery novel, *The Body in the Library* by Agatha Christie, and appeared in the *Saturday Evening Post* (Christie, 1941).

The original illustration shows three figures: Adelaide (Addie) Jefferson, a young widow; Hugo McLean, her old beau; and Mrs. Dolly Bantry, an older woman. The illustration depicts a scene in which Addie has been revealing many of her life's secrets to Dolly, in whose library a body has just been discovered. Addie has just expressed her extreme dislike of the victim, saying "Oh, I could have killed her!" then followed her exclamation with "What an awful thing to say!" Hugo came up quietly behind them and inquired, "What's an awful thing to say?" Addie explained what she had said, and Hugo, who has a romantic interest in Addie, reflected a while and said protectively, "No, wouldn't say that if I were you. Might be misunderstood." He went on to warn her, "You've got to watch your step, Addie" (Christie, 1941, p. 85). The illustration as it appears on the card is cropped so that it only shows two of the figures, Addie and Hugo. The illustration was suggested by Wyatt and was first used in Series C.

Card 7 BM

"A gray-haired man is looking at a younger man who is sullenly staring into space." The original image comes from an advertisement for Fleishmann's yeast that appeared in at least a dozen popular magazines in the fall and winter of 1930 (e.g., "The Whole System Suffers," 1930). The ad was part of a long-running series that featured endorsements by a string of mostly European doctors. They encouraged the use of yeast in the treatment of a variety of physical complaints, including indigestion, headache, constipation, skin problems, and bad breath. The ad under consideration features a distinguished, gray-haired man, the Parisian physician Georges Rosenthal. Rosenthal is pointing out something to a young man, presumably a patient suffering with constipation. The doctor is quoted as saying, "Keep the digestive and intestinal tract clean with fresh yeast and your health will improve" ("The Whole System Suffers," 1930, p. 88). The ad encourages one to eat three cakes of yeast a day. The advertisement bears the copyright 1930 by Standard Brands.

It is not known whether a cropped version of the advertising photo or drawing of it was used in Series A. The picture used in Series B and Series C is clearly a drawn copy of part of the advertising photo. In his redrawing of the picture for Series D, Thal changed the hairstyle of both men and altered the expression of the young man but kept the other features very similar to the earlier drawing and the advertising photo. Thal's original drawing for Card 7 BM can be found at the Institute of Personality and Social Research (Oxford Court Building, 2150 Kittredge St., Berkeley, CA 94720). It was given by Murray to Sanford, who brought it to Berkeley and placed it in storage for many years. When the institute moved to its current address, the picture was framed and mounted for display (R. Helson, personal communication, January 23, 1997).

Card 7 GF

"An older woman is sitting on a sofa close beside a girl, speaking or reading to her. The girl, who holds a doll in her lap, is looking far away." The image on this card is a black and white reproduction of the painting *Fairy Tales* by American artist Anatol Shulkin (1899–1961). Typical of Shulkin's work, the young girl is gazing into space, which according to one critic, allows his models to avoid revealing their inner selves (Bird, 1938).

The painting was purchased by the Metropolitan Museum of Art in December 1938. I have been unable to locate a published color reproduction of the painting, but a black and white reproduction of it can be found in *Art Digest* (Bird, 1938). This painting was suggested for use by Ruesch and was used in Series C.

Card 8 BM

"An adolescent boy looks straight out of the picture. The barrel of a rifle is visible at one side, and in the background is the dim scene of a surgical operation, like a reverie-image." This picture is a drawing by Thal that is based on a color illustration by the American illustrator Carl Mueller (1894–1970). The original illustration was drawn to accompany a short story, "Wild Geese Flying" by Hal Borland, that appeared in *Collier's* (Borland, 1939). The illustration shows Malcolm, a young man, and in the background appears his father, a country doctor, performing an emergency appendectomy on Andy Oliver, a Mexican sheepherder who had threatened to kill his father 3 days earlier. Malcolm assists his father as an anesthetist while another sheepherder watches. It is at this time that Malcolm decides to follow in his father's footsteps and become a doctor. Malcolm's father dies 2 weeks later and leaves him the sum total of his estate consisting of two shotguns and a worn medicine kit.

In the redrawing, Thal gave Malcolm a slightly more youthful and longer face and eliminated his shadowy figure from the background. Thal also omitted the bottom half of the original illustration that reveals a medical bag with a stethoscope and Muller's signature. The gun reminds the reader that Malcolm has been on a goose hunting trip with his terminally ill father when the action in the background took place. The illustration was suggested by Wyatt and was used in Series C.

Card 8 GF

"A young woman sits with her chin in her hand looking off into space." This card presents a reproduction of an oil painting by the American painter Frederic Taubes (1900–1981). The work is titled *Lili, Portrait of the Artist's Wife* and was painted in 1937. The artist's signature can be seen on the card in the lower left quadrant of the painting beneath the chair rail.

The painting is now in the collection of the Metropolitan Museum of

Art in New York City (Taubes, 1937). I have been unable to find a published color reproduction of this painting, but a black and white reproduction of it can be seen in *American Artist* (Hines, 1974). Ruesch recommended this work for inclusion in the TAT, and it was used in Series C.

Card 9 BM

"Four men in overalls are lying on the grass taking it easy." This picture was drawn by Thal from a photograph titled *Siesta,* by the American photographer Ulric Meisel. The photograph shows another man with his hat pulled down lying in the grass, whereas the drawing shows this other man as bare headed. The photograph is more clearly identifiable as western because of the presence of chaps and cowboy hats on the figures. The photograph itself was used as Card 16 M in Series C.

The Meisel photograph was selected for *U.S. Camera—1942* (Maloney, 1941). The caption states that the photo was taken on the 6666 Ranch located near Guthrie, Texas, and was one of a series of pictures taken by Meisel depicting the lives of modern cowboys. According to Meisel, this picture was taken after lunch when the cowboys flopped on the ground to tell yarns, roll cigarettes, and take it easy for a while (Maloney, 1941).

Card 9 GF

"A young woman with a magazine and a purse in her hand looks from behind a tree at another young woman in a party dress running along a beach." This picture is a black and white reproduction of a color illustration by the American illustrator Harry Morse Meyers (1886–1961). It appeared in *Collier's,* accompanying the serialized novel *Appointment in India* by Lawrence Blochman (1940). A chance encounter on a beach near Shakkapur between Virginia Hatton, the attractive sister of a district officer, and Rhoda Curring, the wife of a plantation manager, is shown. Virginia, feeling upset with her thoughts in turmoil, felt the need to take a walk. She strolled aimlessly along the seashore and there observes Rhoda, half running, half walking along the beach toward her own bungalow with her copper-colored hair flying in the wind. The suddenness of her unexpected appearance made Virginia's heart skip a beat. Meyers's signature can be barely seen in the lower left-hand corner of the card (Blochman, 1940). This illustration was suggested by Wyatt and was used in Series C.

Card 10

"A young woman's head [rests] against a man's shoulder." The image appears in substantially the same form in Series B and Series C, but it was redrawn by Thal for Series D. The earlier card appears to be a reproduction of a photograph instead of a drawing and shows the woman's left hand in a slightly different position.

Card 11

"A road [is] skirting a deep chasm between high cliffs. On the road in the distance are obscure figures. Protruding from the rocky wall on one side is the long head and neck of a dragon." When the manual for the 1943 edition of the TAT was printed, it contained a footnote: "Any information leading to the discovery of the originals of Pictures 11 and 20 will be gratefully received" (Murray, 1943, p. 20). In a letter dated November 30, 1943, Rene Spitz responded to Murray's request identifying the painting as *Die Fels-Schlucht* (*The Rocky Gorge*) or *Die Drachenschlucht* (*The Dragon's Ravine*) and the artist as Arnold Boecklin (Spitz, 1943). The manual was then revised to include this information.

This card indeed presents a work by Böcklin (1827–1901), perhaps the best-known 19th-century Swiss artist. The work is titled *Drachen in einer Felsenschlucht* (*Dragon in a Rocky Gorge*). It was painted in 1870 in Basel, Switzerland. I have been unable to locate a published color reproduction of it, but black and white reproductions can be found in *Masters in Art: A Series of Illustrated Monographs* (1906), *Arnold Böcklin* (Schmid, 1919), and *Arnold Böcklin: Die Gemalde* (Andree, 1977).

Once, when Böcklin was crossing the St. Gotthard Pass in the Swiss Alps at night in a very heavy fog and having trouble finding his way, all kinds of unusual fancies came to his mind including *Mignon's Song* by Johann Wolfgang von Goethe.

> Know'st thou the mountain where, hidden in clouds,
> The mule seeks the path which the vapor enshrouds?
> Where horrible dragons in caves rear their broods,
> And rocks uprooted by storms and floods? (*Masters in Art,* 1906, p. 21)

The artist recalled this experience in the painting showing a party of travelers and laden mules in the Alps with night coming on. Suddenly, to their horror, a dragon crawls toward them out of its den. The painting is in the Schack Gallery in Munich, Germany. The picture had previously been used in Series B and Series C.

Card 12 M

"A young man is lying on a couch with his eyes closed. Leaning over him is the gaunt form of an elderly man, his hand stretched above the face of the reclining figure." This image is similar to ones appearing in Series A, Series B, and Series C. It was redrawn by Thal for Series D to show an older man standing by the couch with his knee on the bed rather than sitting in a chair beside the couch. The man lying down is wearing a coat in the earlier picture.

Card 12 F

This is a "portrait of a young woman. A weird old woman with a shawl over her head is grimacing in the background." According to Murray (1943/1971), this drawing was done by Morgan after a painting by the English artist Augustus Edwin John (1878–1961). John produced a number of works with the title, *Strange Companions* (circa 1920–1925; Christie, Manson & Woods, 1963). A black and white reproduction of the one from which this image originated can be found as Plate 17 in *Augustus John* (Bertram, 1923). Morgan's drawing is strikingly similar to this reproduction, except that in the John painting, the young woman on the left is wearing a large bow at her neck. I have thus far been unable to locate a color reproduction of this painting or to find its current location. The image previously appeared in Series B and was not used in Series C.

Card 12 BG

"A rowboat is drawn up on the bank of a woodland stream. There are no human figures in the picture." This photograph by Harold Grainger appears in *Camera Craft* (Grainger, 1937). Grainger, a well-known English writer, lecturer, judge, critic, associate, and later a fellow of the Royal Photographic Society, wrote an extensive series of articles for beginners. After considering two other inferior photographs of the same scene, he argued that this photograph is better because of its feeling of completeness, feeling of harmony, and sense of aerial perspective.

It is of interest that Grainger (1937) went on to present three more photographs of this same general scene. The view he most preferred shows a profusion of daffodil blooms in the immediate foreground in addition to the hawthorne tree, boat, and stream. The boat was in the middle distance rather than the foreground, as in the TAT image. This photograph was suggested by Sanford.

Card 13 MF

"A young man is standing with a downcast head buried in his arm. Behind him is the figure of a woman lying in bed." The image is similar in many respects to one in Series B and was not used in Series C. It was redrawn by Thal for Series D. The earlier picture shows a man standing with his arms at his side, shirt opened, and his full face visible. The table in the earlier picture holds a bottle and an overturned glass instead of the lamp and books. The woman's breasts appear slightly more covered in the earlier picture.

Card 13 B

"A little boy is sitting on the doorstep of a log cabin." According to Murray (1943/1971), this picture is taken from a photograph by Nancy Post Wright titled *Mr. Abe Lincoln, Jr.* Actually the original photograph was taken by the American photographer Marion Post (1910–1990), who was later to use her married name, Marion Post Wolcott. The original photo was captioned, "Old mountain cabin made of hand hewn logs near Jackson, Breathitt County, Kentucky" (*America 1935–1946: The FSA/OWI Photographs,* 1984).

The photograph is dated September 1940 and was taken while the photographer was working on assignment for the Farm Security Administration. The original negative is in the Library of Congress Prints and Photographs Division (Photo LC-USF34–55829-D). A microfiche reproduction can be found in the collection *America 1935–1946: The FSA/OWI Photographs* (1984). The original photograph shows a larger view of the log cabin and has the effect of making the young boy appear smaller and less significant. The cropped and enlarged print used by Murray focuses the attention of the observer on the child, as does the change in title, and makes it easier to relate to the boy.

Murray's misattribution of the photograph is both unfortunate and puzzling in some respects. It is unfortunate because this photograph is likely the most often viewed and most closely examined of any of the photographer's work. It was also arguably one of her best and favorite photographs. It was selected by Edward Steichen to appear in *U.S. Camera— 1942* (Maloney, 1941) and by the photographer herself to appear in *A Vision Shared* (O'Neal, 1976). It is puzzling because although there has been ample confusion in the past concerning the citation of the photographer's work, none have been so far off the mark as was Murray.

A likely source of some of Murray's confusion concerning the photographer's name may have been because of the publication of the picture and caption in *U.S. Camera—1942,* which attributed the photo to Nancy Post Wolcott. It also had the caption of "Mr. Abe Lincoln, Jr.," which is different from the caption in the Farm Security Administration records. The notes in the *U.S. Camera—1942* caption state, "on special assignment for the Farm Security Administration, Mrs. Wolcott photographed this boy as typical of the isolation and meager living of the residents of Breathitt County (Kentucky)" (Maloney, 1941, p. 78). The picture was picked up by at least one newspaper, *The Post Standard* of Syracuse, New York (*Mr. Abe,* 1941). It repeated the name error found in *U.S. Camera—1942. U.S. Camera—1942* is the likely origin of the name change from Marion to Nancy; the change was passed on by Murray because this same issue was likely the source of the image in Card 9 BM (Maloney, 1941). However, it leaves unexplained the other name change of Wolcott to Wright found in Murray (1943/1971).

Card 13 G

"A little girl [is] climbing a winding flight of stairs." This picture is a photograph by Japanese American photographer Hisao E. Kimura (1902– 1975), titled *To Roof Garden*; it appeared in *American Photography* (Kimura, 1934). Murray (1943/1971) was in error, however, when he described the model as "a little girl." The model was Chieko Kimura, the wife of the photographer (S. Kimura, personal communication, April 30, 1993). At the time the photograph was taken, Kimura was an amateur photographer and active member of the Japanese Camera Pictorialists of California in Los Angeles (Reed, 1985). The photograph was suggested by Sanford.

Card 14

"The silhouette of a man (or a woman) [is shown] against a bright window. The rest of the picture is totally black." This drawing by Morgan, another of the old standbys, appeared previously in Series A, Series B, and Series C.

Card 15

"A gaunt man with clinched hands is standing among gravestones." This picture is a reproduction of a woodcut print by the American illustrator and author Lynd Kendall Ward (1905–1985). It appears in his book *Madman's Drum: A Novel in Woodcuts* (Ward, 1930). His novel, the second of six in this genre, consists entirely of woodcut prints, and the "reader" begins to construct the plot as he or she views the prints and turns the pages. The plates and pages of the book are not numbered, but the card is taken from the 116th (third from last) print. It can also be found in *Storyteller Without Words* (Ward, 1974). It should be noted that Murray (1943/1971) gave the date of publication as 1938, although the book was first published in 1930 by Jonathan Cape and Harrison Smith in New York and Jonathan Cape, Limited in London.

Ward (1974) commented that *Madman's Drum* takes place in a foreign country a century or more ago and concerns things that result from universal human relationships. Ward's (1929) first novel, *God's Man: A Novel in Woodcuts,* was better received, perhaps because of the more easily followed story line. E. P., an art critic for *Burlington Magazine,* was of the opinion that this experiment in form was a failure largely because of the conflict in trying to follow the thread of the narrative while also trying to perceive the merits of the pictures (E. P., 1931). The image previously appeared in Series B and Series C.

Card 16

"Blank card" was not included in the set of Series B (Rapaport et al., 1946; White et al., 1941). A blank card was, however, used along with the earliest cards, although references to it are somewhat ambiguous as to whether it was thought to be included as part of the TAT. For example, "the E [experimenter] hands the S [participant] a blank card (the same size as the cards used in the Thematic Apperception Test . . .)" (Murray, 1938, p. 407). A blank card was also used in Series C.

Card 17 BM

"A naked man is clinging to a rope. He is in the act of climbing up or down." Murray (1943/1971) stated that this picture is a drawing by Thal after an unfinished sketch by Honoré Daumier. A French cartoonist, lithographer, and painter, Daumier (1808–1879) did paint a canvas entitled *L'homme à la Corde à Nœuds* (*The Man on a Rope*) in about 1860–1862, during a period described by Rey (1985) as "years of joyless work and discouragement" (p. 38). There are three versions of this composition (Maison, 1968). The earliest version is at the National Gallery of Canada in Ottawa, Ontario. A version at the Museum of Fine Arts in Boston is the second; the final version, nearly a silhouette with knots in the rope, is in a private collection in Paris, France. There is also a pencil drawing of the same model (Klossowski, 1923). The first two versions are unsigned, and Murray (1943/1971) and Holt (1978) have both noted that the source was an unfinished sketch. It is unknown for sure which version was used by Morgan and later redrawn by Thal, but I suspect it was the version acquired by the Museum of Fine Arts in 1943.

The paintings are listed with a subtitle, *Le Badigeonneur—L'évasion* (Maison, 1968). Holt (1978) referred to the title of the source as "The Housepainter." Color reproductions of the Museum of Fine Arts' oil painting can be found in *Honoré Daumier* (Adhémar, 1954; Rey, 1985).

The image first appeared in Series A and is in "Thematic Apperception Test" (Morgan & Murray, 1938). It later appeared in substantially the same form in Series B. It was not used in Series C and was then redrawn by Thal for Series D. Consistent with the Daumier painting, the earlier images show much less facial detail than does the Thal drawing.

Card 17 GF

This card shows "a bridge over water. A female figure leans over the railing. In the background are tall buildings and small figures of men." This picture contains another woodcut from *Madman's Drum* (Ward, 1930). Again, the pages and plates of the book are unnumbered, but the print is the 71st. Another reproduction can be found in *Storyteller Without Words* (Ward, 1974). The image appears earlier in Series B but was not used in Series C.

It is interesting that Ward also recognized what psychologists have referred to as the *projective assumption*. A person's cumulative associations of his or her own experience provide the basis for understanding and attributing meaning to each of the images. The individual who "reads" such a pictorial narrative is thus free to develop his or her own interpretation of the story (Ward, 1974).

Card 18 BM

"A man is clutched from behind by three hands. The figures of his antagonists are invisible." The image, another of the old standbys drawn by

Morgan, was used previously in Series A, Series B, and Series C. However, the earlier descriptions read "a young man helplessly clutched from behind by *two* hands, one on each of his shoulders. The figure of the antagonist is invisible" (emphasis added; Morgan & Murray, 1935, p. 297). The same description of two hands is given in *Morgan–Murray Thematic Appercep-tion Test* (White et al., 1941). By Series C, the description of the card had changed to three hands.

Card 18 GF

"A woman has her hands squeezed around the throat of another woman whom she appears to be pushing backwards across the banister of a stair-way." This image was redrawn by Thal from Series B and was not used in Series C. Holt (personal communication, March 2, 1994) reported hav-ing a vague memory of seeing a photograph from which Morgan drew this earlier picture. In the earlier picture, the woman leaning backward across the banister has on a print dress and the woman with her hands at the other's throat appears to be younger. The stair steps are not visible in the earlier picture.

Card 19

This is "a weird picture of cloud formations overhanging a snow-covered cabin in the country." This picture is a black and white reproduction of a watercolor and gouache painting, *The Night Wind* (Munson-Williams-Proctor Institute, 1970) by American artist Charles Ephriam Burchfield (1893–1967). The work was painted in 1918 and owned by A. Conger Good-year, who granted permission for its use in the TAT (Munson-Williams-Proctor Institute, 1970; Murray, 1943/1971). Color reproductions of *The Night Wind* can be found in "No Place Like Home" (Adams, 1997), *Charles Burchfield* (Baigell, 1976), and *The Paintings of Charles Burchfield* (Ma-ciejunes & Hall, 1997). Later, the painting was given to the Museum of Modern Art in New York City. The painting shows the home of Mrs. Mar-garet "Pommy" Weaver next door to where the artist lived in Salem, Ohio, and recreates a specific childhood impression of monsters and strange phantoms flying over the land (Burchfield, 1930).

On September 22, 1916, Burchfield made a note that seems to presage the painting. In the note, he mentioned a high wind out of the southwest, clouds with black irregular openings that seem like strange creatures above a house with an evil yellow window amid black clawing trees (Town-send, 1993). In that same year, suffering from severe depression and hal-lucinations, Burchfield made some sketches in his notebook, "Conventions for Abstract Thought," in which he developed various symbols from ab-stract shapes for various moods or pathological states including fear, in-sanity, brooding, morbidness, and imbecility. The spiral symbol of fear can be recognized in the gale sweeping across the sky, and the empty-eyed mask of night over the house is recognized as the symbol of imbecility.

Morbidness (evil) can be found in the shape of the windows of the house (Baigell, 1976; Baur, 1956a; Townsend, 1993).

These same symbols can also be seen in a slightly earlier painting *Church Bells Ringing, Rainy Winter Night* from 1917 (Baur, 1956b). These "conventions . . . make it clear that Burchfield was first and foremost a psychological artist—an expressionist and subjectivist, as it were" (Kuspit, 1997, p. 127). Kuspit maintained that fear is the most fundamental emotion in Burchfield's art. In fact, soon after painting *The Night Wind,* Burchfield was drafted into military service for World War 1. *The Night Wind* was suggested by Wyatt.

Card 20

"A dimly illumined figure of a man (or woman) in the dead of night [is] leaning against a lamp post." This image was suggested by Sanford. The following footnote to the description of this card appeared in Murray's (1943/1971) manual:

> Many hours have been spent searching through periodicals and books to find the original of which this is a reproduction. In using it for scientific purposes without the express consent of the artist or publisher we are trusting to their generosity and goodwill, none of our requests for permission to use a picture having been refused by anyone to date. Any information leading to the discovery of the original of Picture [Card] 20 will be gratefully received. (p. 20)

The source of Card 20 is a photograph titled *In the Park* by Dushan (1938) that was published in *Minicam.* The photograph accompanies an article by Dushan in which he urged the photographer to go out in bad weather and take photographs. This particular photo is used to illustrate how haze makes it possible to photograph a light source without causing halation (the spreading of light beyond its proper boundaries in a developed image; Dushan, 1938). The image on Card 20 is cropped significantly at both bottom and top compared with the original, although no important details are omitted.

Concluding Comments

None of the current images on the TAT is entirely original with Series D. Many had been used in the previous series of cards. In addition, it is evident that some of the old standbys drawn by Morgan were not images created by her imagination. Card 1 is taken from a photograph of Y. Menuhin, Card 3 BM is from a photograph of undetermined origin, and Card 12 F is a slight modification of a painting by John. It might be reasonable to speculate that some, if not all, of the remaining images attributed to Morgan also had their ultimate origins in photographs or published pictures. The images attributed to Thal were obtained in a similar manner by redrawing images from other editions of the TAT and a photograph by Meisel. The remaining images were black and white reproductions of paintings, illustrations, or photographs that had been published elsewhere.

Over half of the Series D images were drawn or redrawn by Morgan or Thal, giving this series of cards a coherence that was missing in the earlier series. The fact that all the TAT pictures were in black and white, even though many of the original sources were in color, also contributed to this look.

Quite notable is the relative lack of documentation for the images provided by Murray. Apparently no documentation at all was provided for the earlier series of cards, so the information provided for the Series D cards was clearly an improvement. The initial oversight is perhaps understandable, given the creative thrust of the group at the Harvard Psychological Clinic. Such attention to detail would have likely seemed rather unimportant by comparison and a task that could easily be left for others to complete at a later time.

The modifications in the images over time from ultimate source to Series D image may shed some light on the thinking of the authors. Most often the changes were made in a manner so as to remove detail and complexity and increase ambiguity. Most likely this represented an attempt at increasing the possibility of projective identification. Of course, the end result is a set of cards that has proved to be immensely popular and useful over the past 20 years (Piotrowski & Keller, 1978, 1989; Piotrowski, Sherry, & Keller, 1985; Sweeney, Clarkin, & Fitzgibbon, 1987).

It is difficult to imagine an endeavor to create new TAT cards on the scale of Murray and his colleagues' efforts at the Harvard Psychological Clinic. However, a similar scientific and artistic enterprise in which the stimulating power of new black and white and color cards is compared with that of the current cards would be welcomed.

References

Adams, H. (1997). No place like home: The works of Charles Burchfield. *Smithsonian, 28,* 58–70.

Adhémar, J. (1954). *Honoré Daumier.* Paris, France: Éditions Pierre Tisné.

America 1935–1946: The FSA / OWI photographs. (1984). South fiche [Microfiche] (No. 120, B-11). Teaneck, NJ: Chadwyck-Healy.

Andree, R. (1977). *Arnold Böcklin: Die gemalde* (Kat. 238). Basel, Switzerland: Verlag.

Baigell, M. (1976). *Charles Burchfield.* New York: Watson-Guptill.

Baur, J. I. H. (1956a). *Charles Burchfield.* New York: Macmillan.

Baur, J. I. H. (1956b). Fantasy and symbolism in Charles Burchfield's early watercolors. *Art Quarterly, 19,* 30–40.

Bertram, A. (1923). *Augustus John.* New York: Scribner.

Bird, P. (1938, November 1). The fortnight in New York. *Art Digest,* pp. 22–23.

Blochman, L. G. (1940, April 6). Appointment in India: The fourth of ten parts. *Collier's,* pp. 19, 44, 49–50, 52–54.

Borland, H. (1939, November 5). Wild geese flying. *Collier's,* pp. 15, 25–26, 28–29.

Boswell, P. (1937). American art as it is today. *The Studio, 113,* 4–23.

Burchfield, C. (1930). *Charles Burchfield early watercolors, April 11–April 26, 1930.* New York: Museum of Modern Art.

Carnegie Institute acquires Leon Kroll's "Morning on the cape." (1936, January). *Art Digest,* p. 10.

Christie, A. (1941, June 7). The body in the library: Fifth part of seven. *Saturday Evening Post,* pp. 26–27, 83–86, 90.

Christie, Manson & Woods [Auction house]. (1963). *Catalogue of drawings and paintings from the studio of the late Augustus John, O. M., R. A.* London: Authors.

Clark, R. M. (1944). A method of administering and evaluating the Thematic Apperception Test in group situations. *Genetic Psychology Monographs, 30,* 3–55.

Cronin, A. J. (1935a). *The stars look down.* Boston: Little, Brown.

Cronin, A. J. (1935b, July). The stars look down (Part 1 of 5). *Hearst's International Cosmopolitan,* pp. 66–69, 101–110.

Dushan. (1938, January). Fog—Friend or foe? *Minicam, 1*(5), 14, 18, 23.

Grainger, H. G. (1937). Pictorialism for beginners. Part VIII: The association of parts. *Camera Craft, 44,* 517–524.

Hines, D. C. (1974, July). Frederic Taubes: A retrospective. *American Artist, 38,* 30–35, 65–66.

Holt, R. R. (Ed.). (1946). [Whole issue] (HUGFP 97.43.2, Box 5 of 7). *The T.A.T. Newsletter, 1*(1) [Mimeograph]. Cambridge, MA: Harvard University Archives.

Holt, R. R. (1978). A normative guide to the use of the TAT cards. In *Methods in clinical psychology. Vol. 1: Projective assessment* (pp. 77–122). New York: Plenum.

Jahnke, J., & Morgan, W. G. (1997). A true TAT story. In W. G. Bringmann, H. E. Lück, R. Miller, & C. E. Early (Eds.), *A pictorial history of psychology* (pp. 376–379). Carol Stream, IL: Quintessence.

Kimura, H. E. (1934, January). To roof garden [Photograph]. *American Photography,* p. 11.

Klossowski, E. (1923). *Honoré Daumier* (2nd ed.). Munich, Germany: R. Piper.

Kuspit, D. (1997). Charles Burchfield: Apocalypse now. In N. V. Maciejunes & M. D. Hall (Eds.), *The paintings of Charles Burchfield: North by midwest* (pp. 126–130). New York: Harry N. Abrams.

Lane, J. W. (1937, April). Leon Kroll. *Magazine of Art,* pp. 219–223.

Maciejunes, N. V., & Hall, M. D. (Eds.). (1997). *The paintings of Charles Burchfield: North by midwest.* New York: Harry N. Abrams.

Maison, K. E. (1968). *Honoré Daumier: Catalogue raisonné of the paintings, watercolours and drawings. Vol. I: The paintings* (Plates 174, 175, & 176). Greenwich, CT: New York Graphic Society.

Maloney, T. J. (Ed.). (1941). *U.S. Camera—1942.* New York: Duell, Sloan, & Pearce.

Masters in art: A series of illustrated monographs (Vol. 7). (1906). Boston: Bates & Guild.

Menuhin, M. (1984). *The Menuhin saga: The autobiography of Moshe Menuhin.* London: Sidgwick & Jackson.

Menuhin, Y., & Davis, C. W. (1979). *The music of man.* New York: Methuen.

Morgan, C. D. (1938). Thematic Apperception Test. In H. A. Murray (Ed.), *Explorations in personality: A clinical and experimental study of fifty men of college age* (pp. 673–680). New York: Oxford University Press.

Morgan C. D., & Murray, H. A. (1935). A method for investigating fantasies: The Thematic Apperception Test. *Archives of Neurology and Psychiatry, 34,* 289–306.

Morgan, C. D., & Murray, H. A. (1938). Thematic Apperception Test. In H. A. Murray (Ed.), *Explorations in personality: A clinical and experimental study of fifty men of college age* (pp. 530–545). New York: Oxford University Press.

Mr. Abe Lincoln, Jr. (1941, December 7). [Photograph]. *The Post Standard,* Gravure Section, p. 1.

Munson-Williams-Proctor Institute. (1970). *Charles Burchfield: Catalogue of paintings in public and private collections* (No. 416). Utica, NY: Author.

Murray, H. A. (Ed.). (1938). *Explorations in personality: A clinical and experimental study of fifty men of college age.* New York: Oxford University Press.

Murray, H. A. (1943). *The Thematic Apperception Test: Manual.* Cambridge, MA: Harvard University Press.

Murray, H. A. (1965). Uses of the Thematic Apperception Test. In B. I. Murstein (Ed.), *Handbook of projective techniques* (pp. 425–432). New York: Basic Books.

Murray, H. A. (1971). *Thematic Apperception Test: Manual.* Cambridge, MA: Harvard University Press. (Original work published 1943)

Murstein, B. I. (1972). Normative written TAT responses for a college sample. *Journal of Personality Assessment, 36,* 109–147.

O'Conner, J., Jr. (1935). Patrons art fund purchase. *Carnegie Magazine, 9,* 200–201.

O'Neal, H. (1976). *A vision shared: A classic portrait of America and its people: 1935–1943.* New York: St. Martin's Press.

P., E. (1931). *Madman's drum: A novel in woodcuts* [Review]. *Burlington Magazine, 59,* 98–99.

Piotrowski, C., & Keller, J. W. (1978). Psychological test usage in southeastern outpatient mental health facilities in 1975. *Professional Psychology: Research and Practice, 9,* 63–67.

Piotrowski, C., & Keller, J. W. (1989). Psychological testing in outpatient mental health facilities: A national study. *Professional Psychology: Research and Practice, 20,* 423–425.

Piotrowski, C., Sherry, D., & Keller, J. W. (1985). Psychodiagnostic test usage: A survey of the Society for Personality Assessment. *Journal of Personality Assessment, 49,* 115–119.

Rapaport, D., Gill, M., & Schafer, R. (1946). *Diagnostic psychological testing* (Vol. 2). Chicago: Yearbook.

Rawlings, M. K. (1935a). *Golden apples.* New York: Scribner.

Rawlings, M. K. (1935b, July). Golden apples (Part 4 of 5). *Hearst's International—Cosmopolitan,* pp. 82–94.

Reed, D. (1985). *Japanese photography in America 1920–1940.* Los Angeles, CA: Japanese American Cultural and Community Center, George J. Doizaki Gallery.

Rey, R. (1985). *Honoré Daumier* (N. Guterman, Trans.). New York: Harry N. Abrams.

Rosenzweig, S., & Fleming, E. E. (1949). Apperceptive norms for the Thematic Apperception Test. II: An empirical investigation. *Journal of Personality, 17,* 483–503.

Ryder, G. (1936). America's international awards at the 1935 Carnegie Institute International Exhibition of Modern Paintings, Pittsburgh, PA. *The Studio, 111,* 63–69.

Schmid, H. A. von. (1919). *Arnold Böcklin.* Munich, Germany: Bruckmann.

Spitz, R. A. (1943, November 30). [Letter to Henry A. Murray] (HUGFP 97.43.2, Box 5 of 7). Cambridge, MA: Harvard University Archives.

Sweeney, J. A., Clarkin, J. F., & Fitzgibbon, M. L. (1987). Current practice of psychological assessment. *Professional Psychology: Research and Practice, 18,* 377–380.

Taubes, F. (1937). *Lili, portrait of the artist's wife* [Painting] (ACC 39.168). New York: Metropolitan Museum of Art.

Townsend, J. B. (Ed.). (1993). *Charles Burchfield's journals: The poetry of place.* Albany: State University of New York Press.

Ward, L. (1929). *God's man: A novel in woodcuts.* New York: Cape & Smith.

Ward, L. (1930). *Madman's drum: A novel in woodcuts.* London: Cape.

Ward, L. (1974). *Storyteller without words: The wood engravings of Lynd Ward.* New York: Harry N. Abrams.

Watson, F. (1939). *American painting today.* Washington, DC: American Foundation of Arts.

The whole system suffers. (1930, October). *American Magazine,* pp. 88–89.

White, R. W., Sanford, R. N., Murray, H. A., & Bellak, L. (1941, September). *Morgan–Murray Thematic Apperception Test: Manual of directions* [Mimeograph] (HUGFP 97.43.2, Box 5 of 7). Cambridge, MA: Harvard University Archives.

Williams, H. M. (1940, March 23). Best man's gift. *Collier's,* pp. 12, 50, 52–54.

Part IV

Research and Clinical Applications

7

The Thematic Apperception Test: A Paradise of Psychodynamics

Edwin S. Shneidman

This chapter touches on two picture-thematic instruments, the Thematic Apperception Test (TAT) and the Make-A-Picture-Story (MAPS) Test. From the moment that the first article on the TAT appeared in print (Morgan & Murray, 1935), it had a wonderfully "American" reception. In contrast with the Rorschach technique, which for a long time had essentially one somewhat sacrosanct method for scoring and interpretation, the TAT was somehow felt to be every clinical psychologist's "baby" to raise as he or she wished. On top of Henry A. Murray's genius, there were numerous modifications—picture-thematic tests for children, for African Americans, for handicapped persons, for North Korean prisoners of war, to mention a few. A TAT newsletter—appropriately named the *TATler* and then the *SpecTATor*—could hardly keep up with these modified offerings. For a while, the TAT was such a grand success that Murray himself (in the post-World War 2 heyday of clinical psychology) came to resent being identified as the author of the TAT, as if that were the primary feat he had accomplished in his full life.

First, I provide some personal notes. From the beginning of my work in clinical psychology in the 1940s, the TAT was my favorite psychodiagnostic technique. It has to do with stories, narratives, plot lines, threads, scenarios, themas, scripts, and imaginal productions—almost like short stories and close to literature. If the Rorschach is a paradigm of the individual's perceptual styles, then the TAT is a paradise of the individual's psychodynamics—the strengths and coping capacities as well as interpersonal neurosis and other possible pathologies; indeed, the complexities of human personality that psychologists are supposed to assess.

One day, while I was administering the TAT, the idea occurred to me that it might be useful to separate the figures from the backgrounds and thus permit the participant to choose among the figures (representing the *dramatis personae* of the world), to place them (in whatever combinations) on the background, and then tell a story about the situation that he or she had in large part created. That night I devised the MAPS test (Shneidman, 1947/1988). I listed 21 backgrounds (living room, street scene, doctor's office, bathroom, dream, bridge, bedroom, forest, cave, cemetery, etc.), and a number of different kinds of figures—adults and children of both sexes, animals, and legendary figures—67 in all, as well as a figure location sheet and a figure identification card. I viewed the MAPS test as a little nephew of the avuncular TAT.

Events have a way of concatenating. The MAPS test led to the book *Thematic Test Analysis* (Shneidman, 1951), and editing that book led me to Murray. Murray's ebullient Foreword is the jewel of that book. In that Foreword, Murray (1951) generously wrote

> in the hands of these talented specialists, its [the MAPS test's] utility seems to have been sufficiently demonstrated that I am prompted to suggest that if the testing period must be limited to two hours, a compound TA-MAPS Test might be most efficient. Workers at the Harvard Psychological Clinic have recently noted the same special advantages of the MAPS Test to which several of the participants in this experiment have called attention. (p. x)

Those "special advantages" refer to the fact that the test taker is required to choose and place the figures on each background picture and thus, in part, create the situation to which he or she then tells a story; and the fact that the choice and placement of figures are recorded on a figure location sheet. Thus, the examiner has *objective* data that are reliably amenable (then or later) to interpretation even before the stories are subjected to the examiner's evaluations and interpretations.

The book is essentially a psychological party. ("Would you please participate and discuss a case?"). In this instance, the TAT and MAPS test protocols for one person, John Doe, a 25-year-old man, are the menu; Kenneth B. Little, Walter Joel, and I are the chefs; and the guest list of contributors was culled from lists of nobility in the world of projective thematic tests: Magda Arnold, Betty Aron, Leopold Bellak, Leonard Eron, Reuben Fine, Arthur Hartman, Robert Holt, Shirley Jessor, Walter Joel, Seymour Klebanoff, Sheldon Korchin, Jose Lasaga, Julian Rotter, Helen Sargent, David Shapiro, Percival Symonds, and Ralph K. White.

Thematic Test Analysis focuses on a single case using multiple assessors, each writing about the exact details of his or her way of doing things, including working notes, intuitions, tabulations, tentative inferences, and final comments. The book is a cookbook, not only of ingredients but almost a motion picture of the process of how the stew is brewed. Bolgar's (1952) review of the book in the *Journal of the American Medical Association* began with the following: "This book represents what is probably the most intensive 'psychological dissection' ever performed on a human being" (p. 973).

At this point, I provide a very brief sampling of the raw data: TAT Card 1—sometimes referred to as the young Yehudi Menuhin, seated, looking at a violin on a table before him. Here is what John Doe said:

> This child is sick in bed. He has been given sheet music to study, but instead of the music he has come across a novel that interests him more than music. It is probably an adventure story. He evidently does not fear the chance that his parents will find him thusly occupied as he

seems quite at ease. He seems to be quite a studious type and perhaps regrets missing school, but seems quite occupied with the adventure in the story. The adventure has something to do with ocean or water. He is not too happy though not too sad. His eyes are somewhat blank— the coincidence of reading a book without any eyes or knowing what is in the book without reading it. He disregards the music and falls asleep reading the book. (Shneidman, 1951, p. 13)

By way of comparison and contrast, the following is John Doe's first MAPS test story, his verbatim response to the living room scene. He selected five figures: M-5, a policeman; M-11, a male figure; F-8, a frightened woman; L-6, a disfigured witch; and A-2, a coiled snake.

Well, let's see. Just make up anything I feel like making up? Well, there's been a knock at the door. This housewife (F-8) goes to her door and sees this terrible looking woman (L-6) and recognizes it as her mother. This woman is being followed by a snake (A-2), which is the symbol of what she really is, I suppose. She calls her husband (M-11) who is very indignant at having the old woman come to the door and also the daughter is very indignant because she had told her mother never to come and let the neighbors see her. But her mother told her that I had . . . that she had come because she wants some money to help her son out of a jam. The daughter asked her why she insisted on having the awful looking snake following her. The mother said, "He's the only one I can trust because all snakes don't wear clothes." Then the snake leaves to go into the yard. (Removes A-2.) Meanwhile a cop (M-5) appears. An officer appears at the door. He inquires into the identity of the old woman. The daughter turns to the officer and says "I have never seen this woman before." The mother, of course, is broken-hearted. She says, "I can't help it if my face is this way. It all happened the day you were born. When they were taking me to the hospital, there was an accident and I received both you and a terrible face." The daughter takes out her handbag and says, "Here's five dollars beggar. Now officer, see that she goes." As the old lady leaves, she turns and says, "Before I am through, you'll give me more than money." She exits. (Removes L-6.) The officer inquired if they are sure they don't know the old woman. The daughter replies, "Perhaps I have seen her but I do not want to admit it." The officer says "OK," and leaves. (Removes M-5.) The husband comes over to the wife and says, "I hope I don't have to look forward to the day when you'll get that old and look like that," and quite an argument ensues. During all this time the door has been left open, and the snake slithers in (Adds A-2) and bites them both. As the wife is dying she says, "At least you won't have to see me when I get old," and they both collapse. That's the end of the story. Is that the way? Short stories like that? (Shneidman, 1951, pp. 20, 24)

It was a thrill for me to see the 17 interpretations of those two sets of stories. Every one of them was interesting and made its own special contribution. I was impressed with the amount of agreement among the interpreters and, more important, their agreement with the behavioral data. My general impression was that most of the interpretive arrows were not only on the correct target but rather near the bull's eye. The whole exercise seemed clearly to demonstrate that there was a kernel of intrinsic validity to the clinical interpretation of projective thematic tests. What that specific "something" was, how it works, how it is developed, and how it can be taught and fostered were all questions that remained to be answered, but—and this is the heartening part for clinical psychologists— the several contributions to the single case of John Doe seem to demonstrate its existence. In psychodynamically skilled hands, the TAT (and the MAPS test) seem triumphant.

Abstracts of Thematic Test Analysis

Taken as a whole, the various approaches to thematic test analysis can be divided so as to emphasize (a) elements or aspects of the story and (b) elements or aspects of the characters.

Elements of the Story

Some TAT interpreters (Bellak, Eron, Holt) observed the ways in which the story distorted the physical properties of the TAT pictures, for example, by adding or omitting objects or people or by distorting their commonly perceived nature.

Inasmuch as the participant is instructed to make up a story containing antecedents, present events, and an ending, deviations from this task merit notice (Eron). Other formal aspects of the story considered are its length (Fine) and vocabulary (Fine, Hartman, Holt). Cohesiveness (Fine, Holt, Lasaga), peculiar verbalizations (Holt, Rotter), bizarre ideas (Lasaga), degree to which the plot is unusual or unstructured (Bellak, Fine, Holt, Rotter), use of first person pronouns and of subjectiveness (Sargent)—all these are used primarily to assay characteristics of the participant's thinking style. The levels of the story, such as description, behavior, wish, mood, and so forth, are also of interest (Korchin). The emotional tone of the story is noted (Eron, Rotter). Additionally, the material is classified as autobiographical (Eron, Rotter), wishful, superficial (Rotter), symbolic, or unreal (Eron).

In the individual story, some interpreters (Arnold, Bellak, Holt, Korchin, Lasaga) look for the main theme, such as all the themes of disequilibrium (Eron) in each story. Sequence of themes is studied (Aron) as well as sequence of personal interactions (Joel and Shapiro). Attention is also paid to methods of solving problems (Rotter), to solutions (Klebanoff), and to outcomes (Aron, Bellak, Eron, Fine, Hartman, Holt, Korchin, Sargent).

The stories are also taken together as a whole to make a sequence analysis (Arnold, Rotter), study the frequency of specific themes (Klebanoff, Rotter), or investigate themes and interpersonal relations and discover the dynamic relationships among themes of primary importance (Symonds).

Elements of the Characters

Many elements used for analysis are related to the story characters. The terms in which the characters are described are noted (White). The affects, feelings, or moods of the characters are analyzed (Arnold, Aron, Fine, Sargent), including irrelevant feelings (Sargent), aesthetic, paranoic, guilty, narcissistic, sadistic, and inferiority feelings (Hartman). The characters' needs, press, and threats are examined (Aron, Cox, Holt, Sargent) as well as their values or motivating forces (White). Their actions (Arnold, Lasaga, Sargent) and conflicts (Bellak, Lasaga), interpersonal feelings and relations (Arnold, Fine, Hartman, Joel and Shapiro, Rotter), and specifically their attitudes toward parents or authority (Bellak, Holt). Punishment, attribution or blame, and patterns of need gratification (Bellak) are used, and attention is paid to defenses, such as fantasy and denial (Aron). Inhibition of aggression or sex (Bellak) and flight from experiencing interpersonal feelings (Joel and Shapiro) are also used. Some authors (Bellak, Cox, Holt, Korchin, Sargent) emphasize only the main character.

Types of Approach

All the methods can be subsumed under five categories: normative, hero oriented, intuitive, interpersonal, and perceptual.

Normative

The normative techniques aim primarily at quantifying thematic test interpretation. They are typically tabular and statistical in nature. The basic operation is one of comparing the tabulations derived from the test protocol of the participant under study with the normative data for similar (or different) groups of participants. The general purpose of such techniques is more often personality research than psychodiagnostic service. Four TAT contributors to *Thematic Test Analysis* are identified primarily with the normative approach (Sargent, Eron, Hartman, Klebanoff). For two others (Rotter, Sargent), it is a secondary characteristic of their methods.

Hero Oriented

It is quite understandable that many interpreters of thematic test material would concentrate on the chief protagonist in the stories—this is the essence of the hero-oriented, need–press, or story character analysis method—inasmuch as historically, it is the most important TAT method. These approaches emphasize the story hero or heroine—needs, pressures, and defenses (Aron); feelings and interactions (Fine); characteristics and relations to other story characters (Korchin); and affects and ego activities (Sargent). Other methods, whose primary emphasis is in some other area,

Table 7.1. Thematic Projective Tests Interpretation Areas Outline

Area	Interpretive comment	Summary impression and implication
Pressures, forces, press	"He is pressed by the outside world."	Abstract aspects of the environment, such as fate and the elements, press heavily on him.
Motivations, goals, drives	"There is a desperate but hopeless yearning for love." "One dominant drive is for security."	He wants love from and has a dependent relationship on his parents, which he never gets; he settles for such substitutes as fantasized fame and prestige. Love is conceived of in infantile terms.
Outlooks, attitudes, beliefs	"He seems fatalistically resigned to a rejecting world." "He is very much aware of economic differences among people." "He has an ingrained hopeless pessimism."	He perceives the world as hostile and rejecting. He has a pessimistic outlook in general. He is sensitive to class and economic differences.
Frustrations, conflicts, fears	"His principal conflict is in the sexual area." "His problems are expressed in symbolic form." "He fears social disapproval and censure."	There are deep, intense conflicts around sexuality and around aggression. Conflicts are expressed symbolically, and they markedly disrupt his everyday life patterns.
Affects, feelings, emotions A. General—other than hostility	"His feeling[s] expression is sometimes inappropriate." "He feels depressed." "There is no reason what[so]ever to infer depression."	There is guilt and shame over sexuality and aggression; fear that fantasies and conflicts will become known; considerable depression, anxiety, and a feeling of being rejected.
B. Hostility feelings	"He has an enormous amount of hostility." "His aggressive impulses are both externally and internally directed." "He may not be notably aggressive in his overt behavior."	There are very strong hostility feelings, unacceptable to him, that are rarely expressed overtly. The direction of hostility is both external and internal.

Sexual thought and behavior	"He may have had a number of transitory sexual affairs." "He has never had a stable heterosexual relationship." "He has had homosexual contacts more out of desperation than out of desire."	He has never had a stable heterosexual relationship, inasmuch as this represents incest to him. There is considerable confusion as to his own sex role. Most of his sexual behavior and fantasy is unacceptable to him.
Psychosexual level and development	"[There is] definite immaturity in psychosexual development."	He shows immature psychosexual development; Oedipal relationships are unresolved.
Superego, values, ego ideal	"His Oedipal problems are entirely unresolved." "His ego ideal was delayed in development." "He has a poorly internalized superego." "He has been unable to form a personally meaningful, integrated set of values."	There is lack of interiorization of parental and cultural values. He has been unable to form a personally meaningful set of values to direct him toward positive goals.
Self-control, ego strength, ego capacity	"Ego breakdown is already in process." "[He has] suspicious self-control." "A number of factors may be noted [that] are indicative of ego strength."	There are certain areas of functioning where ego strength is apparent, but ego breakdown is already in process.
Self-concept, insight into self	"He conceives of himself as ill." "He has little hope for his [own] recovery." "He shows some degree of insight."	He considers himself sick and helpless. Generally, there is very little insight in relation to his problems regarding affectional needs.
Personality defenses and mechanisms	"The primary defenses to his conflicts have been withdrawal and fantasy." "[He shows a] patently paranoid form of projective mechanism." "[He has] obsessive defenses."	He uses a variety of defensive mechanisms, with few useful modes of gaining satisfactions. His primary emphasis is on the use of projection and withdrawal. He handles anxiety by avoidance, denial, and use of illness; he reacts to frustration by withdrawal, by aggression against others, and by aggression against himself.
Reality contact, orientation	"There is [a] distortion of perceptual contact with [his] reality." "He has a lessening of the ability to distinguish fantasy from reality." "He is still superficially oriented."	There is a considerable distortion of reality with signs of confusion and disorientation.

Table continues

Table 7.1. (*Continued*)

Area	Interpretative comment	Summary impression and implication
Interpersonal and object relations A. General—other than with parents	"He lacks positive interpersonal relationships." "[He experiences] sibling rivalry conflict[s]." "He has a dichotomous conception of women as either good or bad."	There is no clear pattern of identification with either sex. He has never had adequate relationships with other people. There is considerable sibling rivalry. He sees women as either good or evil.
Attitudes toward—from parents	"His father does not appear to be as important a source of affection as his mother." "He sees [his] father as an inadequate person." "[His] mother is pictured as distant."	He does not identify adequately with either parent but more with his mother than his father. His parents reject him. He fears his mother but is strongly attracted to her; his mother is the more important figure in his life.
Quality of perception, fantasy, language, and thought	"His fantasy life is not well organized." "He often lapses into [an] autistic use of language." "There is a pathologic loosening of orderly thought processes."	There are pathologic thought processes and autistic and contaminated thinking. There is rich fantasy material, but it is loosely organized. There is good but somewhat pretentious vocabulary, with some impairment of his ability to communicate.
Intellect and abilities	"[He shows] at least bright, normal intelligence." "His comprehension is little affected." "[He shows] some creative and literary ability."	Basic intellectual functions are little affected, although there are some deviant intellectual processes. He has many unrealized potentialities. His intelligence level is bright, normal to superior, but with some lowering of actual efficiency because of emotional disturbances.
Symptoms, diagnoses, etiology	"[He seems to be] in early stages of paranoid schizophrenia." "He presents many psychosomatic symptoms."	The diagnosis is schizophrenic or near-schizophrenic reaction, paranoid type, of relatively brief duration. He is a withdrawn individual with delusions, hallucinations, and ideas of reference. He probably acts out his conflicts. He presents some hypochondriacal complaints and possibly shows extreme mood shifts.

Prognoses and predictions, treatment	"His depression is so powerful that suicide is a possibility that must be considered." "The psychotherapy prognosis for him is only fair."	There is a definite suicidal risk and some possibility of homicidal acts. Without therapy, he is likely to become a chronic psychotic. Psychotherapy would be a long-term, difficult process.
Postdictions A. Factual biographical data	"Quite likely he is a member of some minority group." "He probably has had some college training but no degree." "He probably has a younger sibling."	He probably had protracted childhood illnesses. He has a vocational history characterized by a lack of occupational success. He has had some college training. He has siblings.
B. Psychological biographical data	"He was an overprotected child." "As a child, [he] gained much of his satisfactions from reading and daydreaming." "Religion appears to have provided a source of comfort to him."	He was an overprotected child. He made early use of fantasy escapes, such as reading and daydreaming, and of religion.

Note. This table shows salient important psychodynamics elicited by the Thematic Apperception Test (TAT). Interpretative comments and summary impressions and implications are from the 17 psychologists who reviewed the same TAT protocol. From *Thematic Test Analysis* (pp. 298–301), by E. Shneidman (Ed.), 1951, New York: Grune & Stratton. Copyright 1951 reverted to editor. Adapted with permission.

have secondary emphasis on the hero-oriented approach (Arnold, Bellak, Sargent, Eron, Klebanoff, Lasaga, Symonds, White).

Intuitive

The intuitive approach, based on psychoanalytic theory, is the most unstructured of the approaches to the analysis of thematic tests. It uses the insightful empathy of the interpreter; it is a kind of free association of the clinician's unconscious against the backboard of the test protocol. Five contributors to *Thematic Test Analysis* seem to use this approach primarily (Bellak, Holt, Lasaga, Rotter, Symonds). Perhaps all the others use it as a secondary technique.

Interpersonal

The interpersonal approach has three proponents for its use as a primary technique. In the first variation, the interpersonal situations of the characters are analyzed (Arnold); in the second method (Joel and Shapiro), the attention is focused on directed interpersonal feelings—hostility, warmth, and flight—both among the story characters and on the part of the participant toward the characters; and in the third variation (White), the participant's "social perception" of his or her story characters and their interaction with one another are the central aspects of the analysis. The interpersonal approach is a kind of psychodramatic variation in which the interactions of the *dramatis personae* of the thematic drama hold the center of the stage for the interpreter.

Perceptual

The perceptual approach has to do with the so-called "formal" aspects of the participant's production, such as his or her distortions of the visual stimulus of the test materials, idiosyncratic use of language, peculiarities of thought or logic, or loose or queer twists within the story itself. None of the contributors identify this technique as the high, primary mode of approach, although several use it as a secondary technique in some of its aspects (Bellak, Eron, Fine, Hartman, Holt, Lasaga, Rotter, Sargent).

Taking all the TAT reports together, I then designated categories to include all the separate and discrete bits of interpretive information. The TAT interpretation areas outline—citing the 18 categories, representative comments, and composite summary statements—is presented in Table 7.1.

Conclusion

Murray's crusade within psychology was against the constricted vision of those who attempted to foster the notion that the only scientific way to study human beings is one that interdicts the examination of some of their most interesting characteristics, such as the flow of mental processes. Murray told psychologists that statistics, nomothetics, tabulations, and precision are undoubtedly greatly desirable goals when they become suitable (i.e., directly relevant) for one's subject matter but to look for as-yet-unattained concepts just because they are "under the lights where the kudos shine" is rather shortsighted.

Robert W. White (1963) echoed these sentiments: "If we are to learn about our subjects' significant thoughts, feelings, and conceptions of themselves, it is necessary to create conditions that will encourage affective involvement and willing self-disclosure" (p. 12). As a means of inferring the vital secret wishes and unconscious fantasies that participants are not able to communicate directly, a thematic projective test is no less than a magic set of optics without which psychologists have only partial psychological vision.

References

Bolgar, H. (1952). Review of *Thematic test analysis*. *Journal of the American Medical Association, 148*(11), 973–974.

Morgan, C. D., & Murray H. A. (1935). A method for investigating fantasies. *Archives of Neurology and Psychiatry, 34*, 289–306.

Murray, H. A. (1951). Foreword. In E. Shneidman (Ed.), *Thematic test analysis* (pp. ix–x). New York: Grune & Stratton.

Shneidman, E. (1988). *The Make-A-Picture-Story (MAPS) Test*. New York: The Psychological Corporation. (Original work published 1947)

Shneidman, E. (Ed.). (1951). *Thematic test analysis*. New York: Grune & Stratton.

White, R. W. (Ed.). (1963). *The study of lives: Essays on personality in honor of Henry A. Murray*. New York: Atherton.

8

Empiricism and the Thematic Apperception Test: Validity Is the Payoff

Robert R. Holt

During the Thematic Apperception Test's (TAT) half century of existence, many other projective techniques and tests have appeared, may have even had a brief vogue, but have faded away. The TAT remains a part of the relied-on fundamentals of most diagnostic testers, at least of those who use projective tests. Survival in the free market cannot be cited as formal evidence of validity, but it surely attests to the power of the TAT to convince its users that it has clinical usefulness. Even though I have long advocated a hard-headed, skeptical attitude for clinicians and taught it to several generations of clinical students, the skimpiness of this test's formal credentials impresses me less than my own experience of its great value as a source of data for the study of personality. In this way, as in a few others, it resembles dreams and conversation.

My first contact with the TAT was in a seminar at the Harvard Psychological Clinic beginning in 1940. Robert White taught TAT interpretation using psychoanalytically based inference. His constant empirical focus was a quiet lesson in not getting too enchanted with speculations that could not be tested. The following year, I began working with the newly returned Harry Murray as a thesis sponsor and joined other then or future TAT researchers, such as Christiana Morgan, Silvan Tomkins, Leo Bellak, Fritz Wyatt, and Moe (Morris) Stein.

Lessons From Rapaport

A few years later at the Veterans Affairs hospital in Topeka, Kansas, David Rapaport put me through a crash course of training in diagnostic and psychological testing. I then was able to see in TAT stories the effects of psychopathology, premorbid personality, prognostic signs, and indications for treatment—none of which had been at issue with the students I encountered at the Harvard Psychological Clinic.

One great lesson Rapaport taught deserves to be reiterated until every diagnostic tester grasps the point. In the assessment of personality and psychopathology, tests do not exist in the same sense as in classical psychometrics. The aim there was to develop the equivalent of physical measuring instruments, which gave a simple, quantitative result: the amount of a clearly definable substance, process, or other entity. Instead, we psychologists confront people with more or less controlled and structured situations, calling on them to cope with problems or react to stimuli; in doing so, they give us an opportunity to observe their personal, often unique, ways of behaving (in the broad sense, including their communicated thought and affect).

Even when we use an intelligence test, although it was designed to give a quantitative measure of an assumed abstract entity, we waste the patient's and our own time if we do not make full use of the opportunity to observe everything that goes on. The same obsessiveness that makes a patient offer interpretations for many a mean demand for defense of an inkblot, or notice and discuss tiny details of a TAT picture, makes the same respondent embroider the definition of a word; the same exhibitionistic intellectualizing shows up in the ostentatious use of rare words and technical phrases whether the patient is talking about a character in a story, the similarity between two concepts, or the associative route from a stimulus word in the Word Association Test to a response. Likewise, for example, someone who is filled with bitterness toward authority figures may betray it in stories about many TAT cards, not merely Card 6BM or 7BM, in explanations of solutions to the Picture Arrangement subscale of the Wechsler Adult Intelligence Scale, in various movement responses to the Rorschach inkblots, and in his or her enacted relationship to the tester, regardless of the test being administered.

Therefore, Rapaport rejected as misleadingly oversimplified the notion that the TAT gives the tester content and the Rorschach, the structure of personality. He taught a conception of what he called "ego structure" (which has also been called "defensive/coping style") and showed his students how to recognize its manifestations in every part of the battery as well as in interviews and spontaneous written texts. Each type of defensive organization might be adaptive (well compensated) or maladaptive (decompensated) to various degrees, which a tester should recognize. Thus, picking up signs of paranoid style helps to fill in a diagnostic picture as well as the portrait of a personality, but his students learned to recognize how it could be used adaptively in solving certain kinds of problems and to detect signs that it was getting out of hand and causing serious breaches with reality.

Rapaport's teaching method relied heavily on the case method. True, we his students had to read; he expected us to master both volumes of his then just-published *Diagnostic Psychological Testing* (Rapaport, Gill, & Schafer, 1945–1946) and, incidentally, all of the other works referred to in them! Of course, none of us came anywhere near to doing that. In didactic case conferences, we would go over every sentence in a TAT (along with every other test in the battery); with his encouragement, we would offer interpretations, but then we would have to explain and justify them, using the principles learned from his writings and lectures. As more information accumulated with the presentation of all the test material, Rapaport would point out how some interpretive hypotheses would be disconfirmed, whereas others would be supported. Thus, we saw how test interpretation was, in miniature, the application of the scientific method; how our confidence in an inference should grow as it was supported by different *kinds* of data (e.g., story content, formal aspects of the stories, and test behavior); and how intuition must be used but could and ultimately should be explicated.

After all the test data had been discussed, Rapaport would bring together the various threads, showing how they could be combined into a diagnostic formulation. Then, he would summarize the findings of the examining psychiatrist and social worker, giving salient details of life history and symptoms that bore on the tentative conclusions based on the tests, wherever possible. In this respect, Rapaport's method was much like Robert White's. The implicit message is that in the end, tests permit psychologists to make conjectures, which sometimes are well buttressed but which ultimately must be tested against the facts of a life.

Why So Little Progress?

It is somewhat sad to recognize how little progress has been achieved toward making the TAT more easily and generally useful, despite the great hopes of the early years and some success in compiling data on norms (Holt, 1978). Some musings follow on possible reasons for this relative failure—only relative because the TAT lives on and still finds its passionate partisans.

No small part of the problem is the misbegotten heritage of expectations based on the psychometric tradition. The TAT is not a test in the sense of a litmus test or even of a test, for example, of aptitude for law school. The latter, like many "multiphasic" personality tests, is an objectively scored device that yields numbers but no qualitative data. Psychologists know the difference, but unfortunately too many adepts of projective testing conclude that they are thereby freed from all of the constraints and discipline introduced by psychometricians, notably, the obligation to worry about reliability and validity.

To take that position is self-defeating. Precisely because the TAT is a complex method of assessing people, which does not lend itself to the standard rules of thumb about test standards, testers need all the help we can get in minimizing its many sources of error and increasing the validity of our conclusions or judgments based on it. Because psychometricians have thought longer and harder about many of the issues than anyone, we can learn much from them.

Here are a few words about reliability. Its basic point is to guard psychologists against confusing the effects of temporary determinants of test performances with effects brought about by the enduring variables of most interest. If they were trying to measure the emotional state of the moment, then the situation would be reversed: They would want to be able to exclude variance attributable to lasting features of personality to maximize sensitivity to the transitory.

So the main thing is to keep in mind what you are trying to do with the TAT rather than blindly follow some rule of thumb. Conceivably, some aspects could make useful measures of mood; if so, not just researchers on moods would be happy but all of us others who mainly care about assessing personality and psychopathology. By the same token, we need to know as much as we can about the effects of the momentary situation, not just of testing but also the relatively temporary aspects of the tested person's life situation. In one study on which I was a consultant, the TAT was used to follow changes in pregnant women at different stages. Of course, repeated measurement made it easier to pick up what was constant and distinguish it from reactions to the phase of pregnancy.

It is therefore meaningless to ask for a quantitative measure of the TAT's stability. Some aspects of the stories (and of the total test performance) are responsive to temporary determinants in the storyteller and in the setting, although other features are determined by aspects of personality that change slowly. But because, for example, even ideational fluency or the (presumed) effects of infantile traumas do change over the years, the test's validity would be poorer if its measurements of these variables were absolutely invariant.

Reliability often means internal consistency, which also implies a different approach to assessment than the TAT provides. Rigid application of that rule would produce a set of pictures that all drew forth precisely the same kinds of data and allowed for the same range of inferences. How boring that would be for anyone taking the test! The test comes close to providing what one ideally wants: a set of pictures that sample different realms of experience, different kinds of fantasies, and different challenges to defensive and coping strategies, in short, as close as possible to a set of images evoking broadly representative life situations (crises, opportunities, threats, etc.). All of which is the antithesis of internal consistency.

As usual, however, there is something sensible behind the psychometric rule: It is dangerous to base a conclusion on a single datum. The Rapaport approach provides another way to avoid that danger and another kind of redundancy that is less wearing on the one being tested. The notion that a single test, no matter how much it is one's favorite, can suffice for the whole task of assessing a complex human being is foolish fetishism. Because a balanced battery of tests provides a variety of both projective and nonprojective techniques and because psychologists learn to look for signs of the same personological determinants in all of them, we can attain the basic objective behind the principle of requiring adequate internal consistency.

Reliability has another meaning, and the TAT worker has to pay particular attention to it, namely, judge (or scorer) reliability. Because few testers use scoring systems but all of us make judgments, it comes down to an important challenge: How well do different clinicians agree in their interpretation of a TAT story? How curious that such a question is assumed to be asking about a property of the test, when it is clearly aimed at the tester–analyst! Harry Murray once worked intensively with two Radcliffe College undergraduates (Ruth Markmann and Shirley Mitchell), teaching them the need–press system and its application to TAT stories. After some weeks of practice, he presented each of them with a series of stories they had not seen before; each scored them independently using his system. The product–moment coefficients of agreements were all .90 or better. Murray had more sense than to say, "the judge reliability of the TAT is .90." Clearly, the site of the agreement was in the trio of them after their joint experience, and it was specific to Murray's scoring system.

So confronted with any proposed scoring scheme or interpretive method, one should ask "How teachable is it?" To what extent can people learn to apply it as intended from available training materials like a manual?

Scoring System Development

In our research on the selection of physicians for psychiatric training, Lester Luborsky and I decided to try to develop scoring systems for the TAT aimed specifically at predicting competence in psychiatric work. First, we selected, from residents in the Menninger School of Psychiatry (Topeka, KS), those who were considered by their supervisors and one another as the best and the worst. We gave them the TAT (among other instruments), adding Lester's then new pet technique, self-interpretation of the TAT. Then we pored over the data on these known cases, he looking for aspects of content and I for formal aspects that differentiated the better from the worse residents and which seemed to suggest relevant aspects of personality or ability. (Luborsky did the same for self-interpretation.)

Then we added the TAT plus self-interpretation to the battery of tests given to all applicants for two classes of residents, replaced names by arbitrary code numbers and deleted other identifying information, and applied our scoring systems. Luborsky, William R. Morrow, and I did the scoring; we looked at the agreements between each pair of the three of us. For the content manual, agreement on the total score was good: .80, .90, and .91. For the formal aspects, it was much worse: .42, .30, and .23; but a single cue, added toward the end and scored by only one pair (adequacy of the hero), proved surprisingly reliable: .78. The self-interpretation manual was only slightly behind: .71, .71, and .68. ($N = 47$–68; Holt & Luborsky, 1958)

Reliability is nice, but validity is the payoff; here, the results were quite different. No matter who scored it, the content manual's total score had no validity against any of our 10 main criteria (judgments of the residents by their supervisors and one another after a couple of years of training). In the scoring of its author, however, the less reliable scoring manual for formal aspects yielded five validities that were significantly better than zero (although the best was just .28). Only one other judge's scoring yielded a single significant validity, underlining the reliability problem. By the way, the rated adequacy of hero did even better: My scores were correlated significantly with four criterion variables, including .31 with the supervisors' ratings of overall competence, and another judge's scores were valid to the tune of .33 and .30 (against peers' judgments of competence; Ns were between 30 and 53; Holt & Luborsky, 1958).

Later, after I had spent a couple of decades developing a method of scoring Rorschach responses for indications of the primary process and of how well or poorly controlled it is and embodying it in a sizeable scoring manual, Carol Eagle adapted it to the TAT (and dreams). After her experience with using it in her dissertation (Eagle, 1966), I revised and extended it somewhat; it is now a part of a book on the general method (Holt, 1999).

The only data on the scorer reliability of the primary process ("pripro") system as applied to the TAT stories comes from two unpublished dissertations. Eagle (1966) reported the following coefficients, all based on $N = 30$: for total pripro, $r = .93$; for percentage of Level 1 (the most extreme manifestations), $r = .90$; for percentage of formal manifestations, $r = .95$; for mean defense effectiveness (DE), $r = .84$. DE is a rating of the adequacy with which the respondent cushions and makes socially acceptable the emergence of primary process material.

Levin (1973), with $N = 8$, reported $r = .69$ for total pripro; for percentage of Level 1, $r = 1.00$; for mean DE, $r = .59$; for mean demand for defense (the implicit need to defend oneself against the impact of any response), $r = 1.00$. The scoring manual, since revised, should support better reliabilities for percentage of pripro and mean DE.

Conclusion

Most testers do not use any scoring system with the TAT, however, but go directly to inferences about the teller of the stories. They may follow one of the published guides to interpreting thematic materials (e.g., Bellak, 1954; Holt, 1978; Stein, 1948; Tomkins, 1947), but so far as I know, no data exist on how well clinicians can agree on their inferences after having studied any one of these sources. There are some studies of the validity of such inference-based ratings and predictions, but it is virtually impossible to decide to what extent good results may be attributed to the interpretive system as compared to the clinician who used it.

The upshot of this state of affairs is that many people thoughtlessly conclude that the TAT lacks reliability and validity, so they frown on its use. The error is much Macmillan's (1991/1997): He condemned psychoanalytic free association as a worthless way of gathering data about personality because no one has ever demonstrated that it possesses these talismanic virtues. One might as well condemn overt behavior on the same grounds.

Let me not be misunderstood. By that last comparison, I do not mean that the TAT has the face validity of directly observed behavior. Of course, it does provide a sample of such data (called "test behavior"), but for the most part, psychologists rely on inferences about other kinds of behavior, inferences that ultimately have to be validated against observations of those behaviors. If signs of various themes clinicians call "anal" lead them to infer that the storyteller is retentive in a miserly kind of way, the resulting prediction must ultimately be validated against someone's observations of the person in situations where he or she has a chance to act like a miser—even though such observations may not measure up to general psychometric standards of judge reliability.

Thus, the TAT has never gained full academic respectability and never will. Yet to a well-educated psychologist with appropriate talents, it provides uniquely valuable data with which she or he can discover a great deal that is true about a person, especially as part of a battery of tests in a multiform assessment of personality. Long may it wave!

References

Bellak, L. (1954). *The Thematic Apperception Test and the Children's Apperception Test in clinical use*. New York: Grune & Stratton.

Eagle, C. J. (1966). *An investigation of individual differences in the manifestations of primary process*. Unpublished doctoral dissertation, New York University.

Holt, R. R. (1978). *Methods in clinical psychology. Vol. 1: Projective assessment*. New York: Plenum.

Holt, R. R. (1999). *Measuring primary process thinking in clinical data*. Manuscript submitted for publication.

Holt, R. R., & Luborsky, L. (1958). *Personality patterns of psychiatrists* (Vol. 2). Topeka, KS: Menninger Foundation.

Levin, L. A. (1973). Hypnosis and regression-in-the-service-of-the-ego. Doctoral dissertation, Boston University. *Dissertation Abstracts International, 33*(12B), 6083.

Macmillan, M. (1991). *Freud evaluated*. Amsterdam: North-Holland. (2nd, slightly expanded ed., Cambridge, MA: MIT Press, 1997)

Rapaport, D., Gill, M. M., & Schafer, R. (1945–1946). *Diagnostic psychological testing*. Chicago: Yearbook. (Available as rev. ed., R. R. Holt, Ed., New York: International Universities Press, 1968)

Stein, M. I. (1948). *The Thematic Apperception Test: An introductory manual for its clinical use with adult males*. Cambridge, MA: Addison-Wesley.

Tomkins, S. S. (1947). *The Thematic Apperception Test: The theory and technique of interpretation*. New York: Grune & Stratton.

9

Linking Personality and "Scientific" Psychology: The Development of Empirically Derived Thematic Apperception Test Measures

David G. Winter

Morgan and Murray (1935) originally conceived of Thematic Apperception Test (TAT) stories as material to be interpreted rather than "scored." During the 15 years following Morgan and Murray's landmark article, psychologists had analyzed TAT stories in a variety of ways. Many used Murray's (1943) systematic need–press–thema scoring system (e.g., Combs, 1946; Sanford, Adkins, Miller, & Cobb, 1943; also see Stein, 1955), sometimes with adaptations, modifications, or additional scoring categories (e.g., Aron, 1949, 1950). Others introduced different scoring systems or categories (see the 15 different techniques of TAT analysis described in Shneidman, 1951, and Murstein, 1963). For example, Tomkins (1947) scored 10 *vectors* (relationships of a character with an object), 17 levels, 12 conditions, and 6 qualifiers.[1] Some systems are based on TAT content, whereas others focus on the form of the stories or the ancillary reactions of the storyteller. Some involve noting the presence of certain defined categories (with or without actual counting); others involve the use of rating scales. A few rely solely on an intuitive and idiographic synthesis of story synopses, selected key phrases, and the overall trend or sequence of stories (e.g., Arnold, cited in Shneidman, 1951).

Without exception, however, all of these TAT scoring systems were developed by the investigator in a more or less a priori fashion; that is, they were developed on the basis of theoretical considerations or doctrine, general clinical experience, the authority of other writers, or clinical intuition. None was developed in a systematic, empirically based way; although in a few cases, efforts were made to validate certain features of the scoring systems after the fact by comparing two groups, either without

---

[1]With this complex scheme, it took 7 pages to analyze a single TAT story, leading Tomkins (1947) to conclude that "this sample of the application of the scoring scheme may well discourage the reader from ever attempting to score the TAT" (p. 41).

(e.g., Henry's, 1947, comparison of Navaho and Hopi TAT protocols) or with knowledge of the two groups (e.g., Balken & Masserman's, 1940, comparison of TAT stories from groups with different psychopathological diagnoses). As Tomkins (1947) concluded with reference to the proliferation of systems for scoring and interpreting the TAT, "at the moment each investigator is a law unto himself" (p. 5).

Shift to Empirically Defined Scoring Systems[2]

Toward the end of World War 2, the career of David McClelland developed in ways that had a major impact on the use of the TAT in a "scientific" personality psychology. McClelland was an ambitious, tough-minded experimental psychologist trained in the rigorous behaviorism of Clark Hull at Yale University and launched on a productive academic career at Wesleyan University. Although he was familiar with the basic personality theories and questionnaires, he was neither particularly interested in nor sympathetic toward the "soft" emerging field of personality as it was being developed by Murray and others. In 1944, because of the dislocations of the war, he suddenly found himself filling in for Donald MacKinnon, who had studied with Murray at Harvard, and teaching personality psychology at Bryn Mawr College. Drawing on MacKinnon's syllabus, notes, and case material readings, McClelland began to use the TAT.

Returning to Wesleyan after the war, McClelland continued to teach personality and expanded the use of the TAT in his teaching (e.g., the textbook case of "Karl"; see McClelland, 1951, pp. 421–424) and in student research that he advised or supervised (e.g., Baxter, 1947; Natti, 1946). He brought a Bryn Mawr graduate from his personality class to Wesleyan as a research assistant to whom he assigned the task of developing a way to interpret the TAT (McClelland interviews, April 1 and July 11, 1996; Louise Lockwood interview, July 12, 1996). At one point, he was interested in developing a TAT measure of the Oedipus complex, guided by Thorndike's scientific credo that

> if something exists, it exists in some amount and can be measured. . . . If the Oedipus complex exists, you should be able to identify it and code it, and recognize it when you see it in the TAT. (McClelland interview, February 10, 1996)

Experimental Arousal of Motives

In the spring of 1947, McClelland advised John Atkinson (1947) in his Wesleyan senior honors thesis on the relationship between "needs" or mo-

---

[2]The material in this section is from "'Toward a Science of Personality Psychology': David McClelland's Development of Empirically Derived TAT Motive Measures," by D. G. Winter, 1998, *History of Psychology, 1,* 130–153. Copyright 1998 by American Psychological Association. Adapted with permission.

tives and "values." Atkinson's study involved perception rather than apperception; however, because in many important respects it prefigured the later TAT motive arousal techniques (e.g., McClelland & Atkinson, 1948), I review it here in some detail.

For the purpose of measuring motives, Atkinson (1947) recognized that projective techniques were "at present the most promising methods" (p. 53), although "experimental demonstration of its underlying assumption has not yet been accomplished" (p. 55). In his honors thesis, Atkinson proposed to test this assumption through measurement of perception rather than apperception. He adapted Miller's (1939) "subliminal perception" experiment, in which people were asked to perceive and discriminate dimly illuminated geometric figures. If such "projective" responses could be affected by experimentally manipulating hunger—a familiar motive with an agreed-on operational definition, Atkinson reasoned—then the same technique could be used to develop measures of other psychogenic motives.

Atkinson's (1947) participants were 8 Wesleyan students who had volunteered to participate in an extrasensory perception experiment testing whether "abstinence from food would increase an individual's sensitivity to visual stimulus" (p. 59). Three were asked to abstain from eating anything after dinner the evening before, and 5 were asked to eat a large breakfast the morning of the experiment. Thus, at the time of the experiment, the two groups presumably had different levels of hunger or *need food*: hungry after 16 hr versus hungry after 1–2 hr. In the experiment itself, participants were shown a series of 15 slides with pictures projected at very low illumination. (Actually, Atkinson modified Miller's, 1939, procedure, so that all slides after an initial demonstration were blank, thus presuming to measure pure projection instead of subliminal perception.) For each picture, participants were asked to tell what they saw.

Atkinson (1947) found that the 16-hr-hungry group tended to make more responses that suggested a higher *need food*, for example, instrumental or goal *objects* (e.g., egg beater, apple) and *activities* (hunting, eating), food-related *places* (kitchen), and people with feelings of satisfied need. Using a standard experimental manipulation of a classical motivational concept (*n* Food, in Murray's, 1938, terminology), Atkinson succeeded in showing effects on perception. These observed effects could then be taken as an index or measure of the original process or characteristic. In short, Atkinson constructed an experimentally derived measure of the projective expression of a motive.[3] As McClelland later described this method,

> having had a Yale training, I was used to thinking of motives as being aroused, because that's what you did with animals. If I had been a

---

[3]Atkinson's results were consistent with the spirit of the times. The postwar "New Look" movement in perception, for example, held that motives and other personality processes could be shown to affect perceptual and cognitive processes (Blake & Ramsey, 1951; Bruner, 1957).

human psychologist, I would have thought of a motive as a *trait*.
(McClelland interview, February 10, 1996)

Actually, some personality psychologists earlier studied personality processes or characteristics by manipulating them in ways similar to those of Atkinson. For example, Freud (1900/1953) reviewed 19th-century experimental research on dream content in the opening pages of *The Interpretation of Dreams*. In a classic experiment, Murray (1933) showed how aroused fear affects people's judgments of pictures of other people. Similar studies involve the experimental manipulation of ego involvement (Sears, 1937), hunger (Levine, Chein, & Murphy, 1942; Sanford, 1936, 1937), and aggression (Bellak, 1942, 1944). McClelland and Apicella (1945, 1947) manipulated frustration and then observed its effects on behavior, particularly verbal behavior and reminiscence in memory.

The Projective Expression of Needs Research Program

Still, Atkinson's thesis only demonstrates arousal effects on perception rather than on TAT stories or apperception. However, the results led McClelland and his colleagues to develop a systematic program of research on the projective expression of needs in thematic apperception, supported by a grant from the U.S. Office of Naval Research (Atkinson & McClelland, 1948; McClelland & Atkinson, 1948; McClelland, Atkinson, & Clark, 1949; McClelland, Clark, Roby, & Atkinson, 1949). These studies were brought together and elaborated in a monograph, *The Achievement Motive* (McClelland, Atkinson, Clark, & Lowell, 1953).

From Perception to Apperception

The first study in the series (McClelland & Atkinson, 1948) is essentially a replication, with participants from a submarine base, of Atkinson's honors thesis procedure involving people's projection, in their own perception, of an aroused hunger motive.[4] The results, albeit significant, are not striking. Casting around for procedures that would produce more striking results, Atkinson and McClelland decided to use the TAT instead of a perception task. Whereas both McClelland and Atkinson were generally

---

[4]McClelland and Atkinson did introduce a few refinements to the earlier procedure. First, they added an intermediate group, who had eaten an early breakfast so were hungry after 4 hr, thus providing a third data point. Then, instead of telling participants that they were studying the effects of abstinence from food on perception (as Sanford, 1936, 1937, did), they went to extraordinary lengths to disguise the purpose of the experiment. One reason for this change was to distinguish effects of a motive as such from effects of participants' *cognitions* (beliefs about that motive). Thus, people who knew they were participating in an experiment on hunger might (consciously or unconsciously) make up stories full of eating and food or they might (consciously or unconsciously) avoid such stories. In broader terms, this change reflected McClelland's (interview, February 10, 1996) experimental background: "I think that was my animal orientation. I wanted it to be as much like a rat experiment. I wasn't telling them anything."

familiar with the TAT and McClelland had already supervised some research studies using it, the origins of the specific decision to use the TAT
in this research program are not completely clear. The decision must have
been made sometime after March 1947, when McClelland and Atkinson
began testing participants in the original perception study (see McClelland
& Atkinson, 1948, p. 207), and July 1947 when they finished because they
were able to give the TAT right after the perception task to some (but not
all) of the participants in the first study (see p. 643). In an autobiographical essay, McClelland (see 1984a, p. 13) ascribed the decision to a 1946
conversation with G. Richard Wendt, but this seems unlikely because
Wendt had already left Wesleyan 2 years earlier. Atkinson, in contrast,
has a distinct and vivid memory of how they decided to use the TAT:

> We were talking about this first experiment in Dave's [McClelland] of-
> fice. Bob Knapp [a newly hired Wesleyan assistant professor and former
> Murray student] walked [through] from one side to the other, and he
> said, "Why don't you try the TAT," and then walked out the door. (At-
> kinson interview, March 15, 1996)

The TAT results are more interesting and encouraging than the results from the perception studies. As hunger increased from 1 to 4 to 16
hr, food deprivation became a more central thema in the stories. Explicit
need for food increased as well as mention of instrumental activity. Actual
goal activity (i.e., eating), in contrast, decreased. Atkinson and McClelland
(1948) concluded that these results are "the first real data showing how
thematic apperception stories are related to a known condition of the subjects" (p. 653). They immediately discussed the implications of their findings for personality theory:

> For instance, it has been commonly assumed that phantasies serve the
> function of partially gratifying unfulfilled desires. . . . The present data
> clearly indicate that this assumption (which Murray also makes—1938,
> p. 260) is wrong, at least so far as these data are concerned. (p. 653)

This conclusion reflects the crucial methodological insight of the empirical derivation procedure, that is, the ways in which a personality variable is manifest in fantasy, apperception, and verbal content generally
cannot always be forecast in advance but can be studied by experimentally
manipulating the variable in question and observing the resulting changes
in fantasy or verbal content. In later years, McClelland succinctly expressed the logic of this experimental-arousal method for interpreting thematic apperception: "You don't know what it means unless you know what
produces it" (McClelland interview, February 10, 1996). Even Murray
(1958) came to agree that "a psychologist should not rely on any presup-
positions about which TAT variables are likely to be indicative of any personality variable" (p. 190).

During the summer of 1947, McClelland and his colleagues began research to extend the hunger and apperception results to the study of a

psychogenic need, namely, the *achievement motive* (McClelland, Atkinson, et al., 1949; McClelland, Clark, et al., 1949).[5] Here, the purpose was not only to demonstrate that aroused *n* Achievement could affect thematic apperception but also to use these effects to establish a measure of that motive. For his dissertation research at the University of Michigan, Atkinson (1950, 1953) carried out laboratory studies with the new TAT measure. The results of these and other studies were drawn together in *The Achievement Motive* (McClelland et al., 1953).

Further Developments of the Empirical Derivation Method

Over the past 4 decades, the idea of using experimental arousal of personality variables and empirical derivation of TAT-scoring categories has been developed and expanded in several different directions (see Smith, 1992b).

Achievement Motivation Research

First, extensive laboratory and field studies of the achievement motive, using the TAT measure, show how the motive is expressed in achieving behavior (Atkinson & Feather, 1966) and how its verbal and behavioral expression fluctuates (in Murray's, 1938, terms, how its "regnancy" varies) in the stream of behavior, as a function of arousing cues and consummatory responses (Atkinson, Bongort, & Price, 1977). This, in turn, has led to a deeper understanding of the apperceptive process itself (Atkinson, 1982), including the issue of TAT reliability (Lundy, 1985; Winter & Stewart, 1977).

Proceeding in a very different direction and at a different level of analysis, McClelland (1961; see also McClelland & Winter, 1969) used a variety of research techniques and interventions to explore economic development as a major social consequence of achievement motivation.[6]

Measuring Other Motives

Following in the tradition of research on achievement motive, researchers designed similar experiments to arouse and measure other motives. Atkinson, Heyns, and Veroff (1954; see also Koestner & McClelland, 1992) used participation in group sociometric ratings as a way of arousing the

---

[5]McClelland and his colleagues described this motive using a variety of names, such as "ego-involvement" and "mastery." As McClelland recalled, "we called it 'mastery' at first. I didn't like 'achievement' because it was too general, but 'mastery' sounded too much like power" (McClelland interview, February 10, 1996; see also McClelland, 1961, p. 301).

[6]Winter's (1991) adaptation of the TAT-based motive scoring systems for use with other kinds of verbal material, including interviews, speeches, popular literature, folktales, corporate annual reports, and diplomatic documents, has facilitated this expansion of personality research well beyond the confines of the psychological clinic or laboratory.

affiliation motive (*n* Affiliation). McAdams (1982, 1992) used a variety of procedures to arouse the intimacy motive, a less defensive and more "sharing" variant of *n* Affiliation. Finally, Weinberger and McLeod (1989) developed a measure of yet another affiliation-related motivational concept, the "need to belong," by comparing TAT stories of people who had been subliminally exposed to the cue "mommy and I are one" (see Silverman, Lachmann, & Milich, 1982; and Weinberger & Silverman, 1990) and people exposed to the neutral cue "people are walking."

Several different investigators have tried to arouse the power motive. Veroff (1957) originally used contrasting groups (candidates for student government awaiting election results vs. students in an introductory psychology class) instead of a random assignment to experimentally aroused and neutral conditions. Uleman (1966, 1972) and Winter (1973), in contrast, used a variety of experimental arousal procedures, such as observing a hypnotist or viewing a film of President John F. Kennedy's 1961 inaugural address. Winter (1973) integrated all of the different scoring systems into a single revised measure of the power motive (*n* Power). Research at the social level suggests that war and peace may result in part from high levels of power motivation and low levels of affiliation (McClelland, 1975; Winter, 1993).

Empirically Derived Measures of Other Personality Variables

Researchers also used empirical derivation to develop thematic apperceptive measures of other personality variables besides motives (see Smith, 1992b). For example, Fleming and Horner (1992) conceptualized fear of success as an ambivalent orientation toward success that is particularly salient for women when competing with men. Using a task labeled "memory and intellectual productivity—arithmetic problems," they experimentally aroused fear of success by directly pairing women with men and giving them success feedback. Women in the neutral group were not paired or given feedback and were told that the experimenters were only gathering norms on the test itself.

Stewart and Winter (1974) conceptualized self-definition (vs. social definition) as a personal style of independence from identity and role prescriptions imposed by others. By comparing college women who planned careers in what were at the time male-dominated fields with women planning no careers, they developed a thematic apperception measure that reflects a generalized instrumental coping style (Stewart, 1992).

Stewart (1982) also used the contrasting-groups technique to develop an empirically derived measure of psychological stances of adaptation, based on the developmental "stages" of Sigmund Freud and Erik Erikson. In subsequent research, this measure has been shown to play an important role in how people adapt to a variety of major life changes (Stewart & Healy, 1992).

Winter (1992b; Winter & Barenbaum, 1985) developed a measure of responsibility that moderates the effect of power motivation by comparing

TAT stories of college students who had younger siblings and had been assigned, as children, major chores, such as child care or food preparation (presumed high responsibility), with those of college students with no younger siblings and no assigned major chores (presumed low responsibility).

By showing a film of Mother Teresa giving aid and comfort to orphans and then contrasting the TAT stories of people whose immune system functioning increased afterward versus those whose immune functioning decreased, McKay (1992) developed a measure of affiliative trust–mistrust. This measure appears to reflect thoughts about relationships and is conceptually related to (although different from) the affiliation and intimacy motive measures of desire or preference for such relationships.

Clearly, then, the spring 1947 decision by McClelland and Atkinson to measure motives by experimental arousal and thematic apperception was a major landmark in the development of scientific research on personality. The decision helps to broaden the use of the TAT from an individualized technique of clinical assessment to a research instrument that could be used in large-scale, group-based research—and further for use in surveys (Veroff, 1992) and archival studies (Winter, 1992a). It also provides an empirically based alternative to a priori scoring systems, making it possible to specify the validity of TAT scoring definitions in terms of precise operational antecedent manipulations.

Comparison of the Murray and McClelland Approaches to Thematic Apperception

The major differences between Murray's original TAT administration and interpretation methods and the empirical derivation methods introduced by McClelland and his colleagues can be summarized under several categories.

Selection of Pictures

Researchers of the McClelland–Atkinson tradition generally do not use the original Murray TAT pictures but rather pictures that suggest more "everyday" situations and that are less emotionally evocative (see Atkinson, 1958, pp. 831–836; and Smith, 1992a, pp. 631–647). For example, Atkinson (interview, March 15, 1996) recalled cutting pictures out of the *Saturday Evening Post* (a popular magazine of the time) for the original achievement motivation study. McClelland discussed the decision to use new pictures along with some of the original Murray pictures in the first TAT study of hunger (Atkinson & McClelland, 1948):

> There were very few Murray pictures that were in any way related to food. They were clearly designed to get at complexes and deep clinical [issues]. . . . We wanted stuff that at least vaguely suggested food so

they could write a story either one way or the other, about food or not.
. . . The main thing [however] was not to make it so much like food that
all the stories would be the same. (McClelland interview, February 10,
1996)

Group Versus Individual Administration

Atkinson and McClelland (1948) administered the TAT to groups instead
of individuals, which meant that participants wrote stories instead of telling them (see also Clark, 1944; and Lindzey & Heinemann, 1955). They
were allowed only 5 min (vs. an unlimited time) per story. Along with the
change of pictures, these changes tend to reduce the emotional intensity
and level of unconscious or primary process in the resulting stories. Although these changes were necessary for reasons of time and money,
McClelland (interview, February 10, 1996) also preferred them on grounds
of its greater scientific objectivity: "I didn't want a personal relationship
between the tester and testee to develop. I wanted it to be like an experiment, in which all people would have the same cues."

Development of a Scoring System

As suggested throughout this chapter, the major difference between Murray's and McClelland's systems involves measurement. Murray preferred
an observer's ratings (individual ratings or pooled experts' ratings) of TAT
stories, behavior, or entire assessment batteries, whereas McClelland preferred objectively defined measures, preferably based on experimental or
empirical derivation, involving only decisions about presence versus absence:

> He [Murray] was wanting always to infer [motives from averaged be-
> haviors], and I didn't want to infer, because I felt different people would
> infer different things from the same behaviors. It didn't seem to me
> that that was science. (McClelland interview, February 10, 1996)

Most of the early TAT scoring systems, including Murray's original
one, were based on theoretical or a priori notions of what should be scored
for what categories. In contrast, the Atkinson–McClelland TAT scoring
system for hunger (as well as most of the later empirically derived scoring
systems) proceeds partly on theory, partly on the basis of logic, and very
much on sheer empiricism—differences between an aroused and neutral
group or between criterion and control groups.[7] As McClelland later recalled, "the empirical difference between the 1-hour and 16-hour TATs was
the main thing. Obviously you didn't look for [just] anything; it had to be

---

[7]As an illustrative example of this procedure, Winter (1973, chap. 3) gave a detailed
step-by-step account of how the power motive scoring system was empirically derived from
aroused and neutral TAT stories and then cross-validated blindly on additional aroused and
neutral stories.

theoretically relevant to hunger" (McClelland interview, February 10, 1996).

Simplified Scoring Versus Ratings

Scoring systems developed in the McClelland tradition of empirical derivation are generally atomistic and simple; that is, they consist of a series of discrete categories scored as present or absent instead of the rating scales (often complex and multidimensional) used by Murray and others. McClelland proceeded, in other words, on the assumption that *extensivity* (scoring many subcategories) is the equivalent of *intensity* (a very strong motive). McClelland (1957) defended his preference for atomistic simplicity over complexity on similar grounds:

> It is precisely because the judge synthesizes many unknown factors in his judgment, that the estimate he makes, no matter how precise or quantitative it may be, is practically useless as far as the development of basic science is concerned. . . . A simple count of frequency at least gives us an objective measure of something which is not a hopeless mixture of a variety of unknown cues to which the judges are responding, plus a variety of personal and cultural factors influencing this judgment. (pp. 375–376)

In later years, McClelland (interview, February 10, 1996) gave additional reasons for preferring this "principle of simplified scoring"[8]:

> I had always found that different judges used different parts of the rating scale. . . . I was also influenced by some work I had done on the Bernreuter Personality Inventory [McClelland, 1944]. [It] had this elaborate weighting system, and I found that simple yes/no's correlated .97 [with weighted scores].

Specification of Motive Arousal Conditions

The decision to define motive scoring systems by experimental arousal of the motive immediately leads the researcher to the problem of deciding how to arouse the motive. How does one know that any particular procedure "really" arouses, for example, the achievement motive rather than the curiosity motive or even the power motive? Alternatively, perhaps these are not three separate motives but rather three facets of one complex motive? In the empiricist spirit, these questions are answered, in the McClelland–Atkinson approach, by grouping together those arousal conditions that produce similar shifts in thematic apperception content (see the footnote on p. 39, Winter, 1973). Thus, two conditions are said to arouse the same motive if they produce the same kinds of thematic apperception; therefore, any particular procedure can be said to arouse Mo-

---

[8]See also Winter (1982, pp. xxv–xxix).

tive X if it produces the same kinds of thematic apperception content as do other Motive X arousal procedures.

McClelland later commented on how this principle—of grouping together arousal conditions that had similar effects on thematic apperception—emerged from early work on the achievement motive. A success-arousal condition was expected to give results that would contrast with those of failure arousal (see McClelland, Atkinson, et al., 1949; and McClelland, Clark, et al., 1949):

> [When] we got into the ego-involvement area[,] . . . we did both success and failure. They came out almost the same. Failure was supposed to be deprivation, but success was almost as good. [We tried success] because it is the opposite of failure, and we wanted to see if it would decrease [achievement imagery]. But it didn't. (McClelland interview, February 10, 1996)

In consequence, both success and failure (along with several other conditions) are considered to be achievement-arousing conditions. Correspondingly, conditions that are conceptually related to a variable and therefore might be expected to produce similar results but do not (e.g., an ego-arousing condition that only elicited inhibited stories; see McClelland, Atkinson, Clark, & Lowell, 1953, pp. 103, 211) are not considered to have aroused the same motive.

Emphasis on Interscorer Reliability

From the beginning, McClelland and his colleagues were concerned with achieving high levels of interscorer agreement—much higher levels than those reported for the early TAT scoring systems. The initial hunger study describes how both experimenters independently scored all stories at first, achieving agreement on 75–80% of classifications. Subsequent discussions led to sharper definition of hazy categories, "so that there was ready agreement on practically all classifications, once the definitions were fully understood by both judges in the same way" (Atkinson & McClelland, 1948, p. 647). The first *n* Achievement study reported even more extensive procedures and data about interscorer reliability (see McClelland, Clark, et al., 1949, pp. 249–250). Over the years, the requirement of high interscorer reliability (typically category agreement of 85% or higher and total score correlations of .85 or higher) has been a consistent hallmark of research carried out with all measures developed in the McClelland–Atkinson tradition. Lengthy scoring manuals and elaborate training procedures were developed to facilitate interscorer agreement (see Atkinson, 1958; and Smith, 1992b).

Conceptual Status of the Motive Concept

Both Murray and McClelland conceived of motives as enduring personality dispositions that are nevertheless subject to fluctuation in salience (in

Murray's terms, regnancy) over time, although McClelland and Atkinson were each concerned, in different ways, with justifying this equivalence. The McClelland–Atkinson technique actually defines motives by arousal-induced changes in thematic apperception. That is, an enduring disposition is defined by state changes. Thus, the technique assumes the equivalence of the state and trait manifestations of a motive—an assumption that was recognized in the very first achievement motivation article: "It must of course still be shown that the situationally induced need affects apperception in the same way as a strong character need would, as clinically or otherwise defined" (McClelland, Clark, et al., 1949, p. 252). In later years, Atkinson (1982; see also Atkinson et al., 1977) developed an elaborate theoretical model that could account for such equivalence.

Empirical Validation of Motive Scores

Both Murray and McClelland assumed that their TAT-based motive measures would be valid in the sense of predicting significant and important real-world behaviors and life outcomes. For Murray and the authors of other earlier TAT scoring systems, however, this assumption was confirmed mostly in clinical practice and with individual cases, if at all. In contrast, decades of systematic research studies contribute to the validity of the experimentally derived measures of n Achievement and other TAT motives measured in this tradition (see summaries by Smith, 1992b; and Winter, 1996, chap. 5). For example, n Achievement tends to predict entrepreneurial behavior and economic success, n Intimacy predicts overall life adjustment, and n Power predicts organizational leadership and having careers with direct impact on other people.

However, personality psychologists in the psychometric tradition are often critical of the validity and other psychometric credentials of the thematic apperceptive measures (see Entwisle, 1972; and Fineman, 1977). There are two reasons for this discrepancy. First, the TAT-based measures are sometimes said to have low internal consistency and test–retest reliability. Several studies (Lundy, 1985; Winter & Stewart, 1977) show that low test–retest correlations are largely an artifact of implicit retest instructions. Atkinson (1982) elaborated his model of the dynamics of action to show how the TAT measures could have low internal consistency yet be valid measures of an enduring disposition (see also Fleming, 1982).

Second, the TAT-based measures have never correlated with self-report or questionnaire measures purporting to measure the "same" motive (deCharms, Morrison, Reitman, & McClelland, 1955; McClelland, 1980; McClelland, Koestner, & Weinberger, 1989; Weinberger & McClelland, 1990). Because of the influence of the multitrait–multimethod principle of Campbell and Fiske (1959) and because questionnaires are quicker and easier to administer and score, many personality psychologists have therefore dismissed the TAT-based measures. However, the multitrait–multimethod principle can be "turned on its head" to argue that two measures of truly different constructs should not highly intercorrelate. Reviewing the literature, McClelland and his colleagues (McClelland et al., 1989; Weinberger & McClelland, 1990) suggested that the TAT-based measures and self-report measures actually reflect different kinds of motives or different motivational systems and should, therefore, not be expected to be highly related to each other.

Creativity in Murray and McClelland: Some Conclusions

Although there are certainly many differences between Morgan and Murray's (1935) development of the TAT as an innovation in personality assessment and McClelland's later transformation of the TAT into an instrument of scientific personality research, both were clearly innovations in personality psychology. From their two contrasting stories, it is perhaps possible to extract some more general conclusions about scientific innovation and the conditions that foster it.

Crossing Boundaries

In both Murray's and McClelland's cases, extrinsic factors play an important role in scientific innovation. Consider their academic origins: Neither started out as a personality psychologist; in crossing disciplinary boundaries, each enriched personality psychology with the perspectives, methods, and concerns of his other field. Murray crossed and recrossed many boundaries—psychology, chemistry, biology, medicine, literature, and culture. From his studies of physiology and medicine, Murray brought with him into personality the importance of a comprehensive catalog of variables, multiple ways of measuring concepts, and an integrative or organismic perspective. His extensive interest and background in literature (see Anderson, chap. 3; and Gieser & Morgan, chap. 5, this volume) may even have prepared him to elaborate, with Christiana Morgan, the principles of the TAT from the germinal experiences and ideas of Cecelia Roberts (see Anderson, 1990, p. 321; and chap. 3, this volume).

McClelland came to personality psychology and the TAT directly from the rigorous tradition of Yale University behaviorism and brought with him many of the principles of that background. Indirectly, his strong liberal arts and humanities background helped to steer his scientific interests in the direction of "humanistic" personality psychology.

The history of personality psychology has many other examples of crossing disciplinary boundaries: Sigmund Freud started out as a physician and neurologist, George Kelly became a psychologist after aeronautical engineering and teaching public speaking, Carl Rogers enrolled in a theological seminary before he realized that his true interest was psychotherapy, Erik Erikson began as an artist, Robert White taught history, and even B. F. Skinner originally wanted to be a writer.

Problems in Crossing Boundaries

Crossing boundaries may facilitate innovation, but it does not always ensure a warm reception or comfortable life for the boundary crosser. Those
in the new field often view such "immigrants" as uncouth intruders; those
in the old field may see them as renegades because boundary crossers do
not fully accept either canon or consistently play by either set of rules.

Murray experienced a good deal of controversy, criticism, and difficulty
on account of his boundary crossings—most notably in his relations with
the rest of Harvard University's Psychology Department and in the dis-
putes surrounding his tenure case (see Robinson, 1993; Stein & Gieser,
chap. 2, this volume; and Triplet, 1983).

McClelland tried to bridge "The Two Disciplines of Scientific Psychology," as Cronbach (1957) entitled his article. Personality psychologists
have always been concerned with the correlation, consistency, and conver-
gence of characteristics that represent individual differences. Experimental psychologists, in contrast, have stressed the importance of manipulation of variables and operational definitions. Any attempt to blend
these two approaches, such as measuring individual differences through
carefully defined manipulation of experimental conditions, thus runs the
danger of alienating partisans of both approaches. Thus, McClelland did
not always win the approval of either field. In later years, McClelland
(1984b) observed that

> perhaps [the problem with the TAT method] is the unusual sensitivity
> of the method to disturbances [or] the time and trouble it takes to learn
> a coding system. . . . [This] did not impress me because I knew that
> biologists were extremely careful in standardizing conditions for taking
> a measurement and would also spend hours making a single assay.
> Why couldn't psychologists take the same amount of trouble? My hope
> had always been that psychologists would see that the [TAT-based]
> method was so valuable that they would use it to develop measures . . .
> of their own. Instead they have put tremendous time and energy into
> trying to find short-cut methods . . . through questionnaires. (p. 450)

Freedom of the "Nonmainstream"

Finally, both Murray and McClelland were able to bring about their innovations because of a certain freedom—freedom from the demands of
both mainstream personality psychology and mainstream academic institutions. For Murray, a certain amount of independent wealth and generous, relatively unrestricted support from the Rockefeller Foundation was
critical to his explorations in personality (see Robinson, 1993). For Mc-
Clelland, the freedom implied by Wesleyan's simultaneous commitments
to excellence in interdisciplinary liberal arts undergraduate education and
in research probably freed him from pressures toward orthodox mainstream research to get tenure. The U.S. Office of Naval Research's policy
of funding basic research was also critical. With the freedom to wander off
on strange paths and to take some chances, Murray and McClelland were

both able to cross boundaries and take risks, thereby discovering new perspectives and innovative techniques.

References

Anderson, J. W. (1990). The life of Henry A. Murray: 1893–1988. In A. I. Rabin, R. A. Zucker, R. A. Emmons, & S. Frank (Eds.), *Studying persons and lives* (pp. 304–334). New York: Springer.

Aron, B. (1949). *A manual for analysis of the Thematic Apperception Test.* Berkeley, CA: Berg.

Aron, B. (1950). The Thematic Apperception Test in the study of prejudiced and unprejudiced individuals. In T. W. Adorno, E. Frenkel-Brunswik, D. J. Levinson, & R. N. Sanford (Ed.), *The authoritarian personality* (pp. 489–544). New York: Harper & Row.

Atkinson, J. W. (1947). *The functional relationship between an individual's needs and his values.* Unpublished honors thesis, Wesleyan University.

Atkinson, J. W. (1950). *Studies in projective measurement of achievement motivation.* Unpublished doctoral dissertation, University of Michigan.

Atkinson, J. W. (1953). The achievement motive and recall of interrupted tasks. *Journal of Experimental Psychology, 46,* 381–390.

Atkinson, J. W. (Ed.). (1958). *Motives in fantasy, action, and society.* Princeton, NJ: Van Nostrand.

Atkinson, J. W. (1982). Motivational determinants of thematic apperception. In A. J. Stewart (Ed.), *Motivation and society* (pp. 3–40). San Francisco: Jossey-Bass.

Atkinson, J. W., Bongort, K., & Price, L. H. (1977). Explorations using computer simulation to comprehend thematic apperceptive measurement of motivation. *Motivation and Emotion, 1,* 1–27.

Atkinson, J. W., & Feather, N. T. (1966). *A theory of achievement motivation.* New York: Wiley.

Atkinson, J. W., Heyns, R. W., & Veroff, J. (1954). The effect of experimental arousal of the affiliation motive on thematic apperception. *Journal of Abnormal and Social Psychology, 49,* 405–410.

Atkinson, J. W., & McClelland, D. C. (1948). The projective expression of needs. I: The effects of different intensities of the hunger drive on thematic apperception. *Journal of Experimental Psychology, 38,* 643–658.

Balken, E. R., & Masserman, J. H. (1940). The language of fantasy. III: The language of the fantasies of patients with conversion hysteria, anxiety state, and obsessive–compulsive neurosis. *Journal of Psychology, 10,* 75–86.

Baxter, C. G. (1947). *Personality and projective techniques: An experimental study of certain aspects of the Thematic Apperception Test.* Unpublished honors thesis, Wesleyan University.

Bellak, L. (1942). An experimental investigation of projection. *Psychological Bulletin, 39,* 489–490.

Bellak, L. (1944). The concept of projection. *Psychiatry, 7,* 353–370.

Blake, R. R., & Ramsey, G. V. (1951). *Perception: An approach to personality.* New York: Ronald Press.

Bruner, J. S. (1957). On perceptual readiness. *Psychological Review, 64,* 123–152.

Campbell, D. T., & Fiske, D. (1959). Convergent and discriminant validation by the multitrait–multimethod matrix. *Psychological Bulletin, 56,* 81–105.

Clark, R. M. (1944). A method of administering and evaluating the Thematic Apperception Test in a group situation. *Genetic Psychology Monographs, 30,* 3–55.

Combs, A. W. (1946). A method of analysis for the Thematic Apperception Test and autobiography. *Journal of Clinical Psychology, 2,* 167–174.

Cronbach, L. J. (1957). The two disciplines of scientific psychology. *American Psychologist, 12,* 671–684.

122   DAVID G. WINTER

deCharms, R., Morrison, H. W., Reitman, W., & McClelland, D. C. (1955). Behavioral correlates of directly and indirectly measured achievement motivation. In D. C. McClelland (Ed.), *Studies in motivation* (pp. 414–423). New York: Appleton-Century-Crofts.

Entwisle, D. R. (1972). To dispel fantasies about fantasy-based measures of achievement motivation. *Psychological Bulletin, 83,* 1131–1153.

Fineman, S. (1977). The achievement motive construct and its measurement: Where are we now? *British Journal of Psychology, 68,* 1–22.

Fleming, J. (1982). Projective and psychometric approaches to measurement: The case of fear of success. In A. J. Stewart (Ed.), *Motivation and personality* (pp. 63–96). San Francisco: Jossey-Bass.

Fleming, J., & Horner, M. S. (1992). The motive to avoid success. In C. P. Smith (Ed.), *Motivation and personality: Handbook of thematic content analysis* (pp. 179–189). New York: Cambridge University Press.

Freud, S. (1953). The interpretation of dreams. In J. Strachey (Ed. & Trans.), *The standard edition of the complete psychological works of Sigmund Freud* (Vol. 4–5, pp. 1–627). London: Hogarth Press. (Original work published 1900)

Henry, W. E. (1947). The thematic apperception technique in the study of culture–personality relations. *Genetic Psychology Monographs, 35,* 1–134.

Koestner, R., & McClelland, D. C. (1992). The affiliation motive. In C. P. Smith (Ed.), *Motivation and personality: Handbook of thematic content analysis* (pp. 205–210). New York: Cambridge University Press.

Levine, R., Chein, I., & Murphy, G. (1942). The relation of the intensity of a need to the amount of perceptual distortion: A preliminary report. *Journal of Psychology, 13,* 283–293.

Lindzey, G., & Heinemann, S. H. (1955). Thematic Apperception Test: Individual and group administration. *Journal of Personality, 24,* 34–55.

Lundy, A. (1985). The reliability of the Thematic Apperception Test. *Journal of Personality Assessment, 49,* 141–145.

McAdams, D. P. (1982). Intimacy motivation. In A. J. Stewart (Ed.), *Motivation and society* (pp. 133–171). San Francisco: Jossey-Bass.

McAdams, D. P. (1992). The intimacy motive. In C. P. Smith (Ed.), *Motivation and personality: Handbook of thematic content analysis* (pp. 224–228). New York: Cambridge University Press.

McClelland, D. C. (1944). Simplified scoring of the Bernreuter Personality Inventory. *Journal of Applied Psychology, 28,* 414–419.

McClelland, D. C. (1951). *Personality.* New York: Holt, Rinehart, & Winston.

McClelland, D. C. (1957). Toward a science of personality psychology. In H. P. David & H. von Bracken (Eds.), *Perspectives in personality theory* (pp. 355–382). New York: Basic Books.

McClelland, D. C. (1961). *The achieving society.* Princeton, NJ: Van Nostrand.

McClelland, D. C. (1975). *Power: The inner experience.* New York: Irvington.

McClelland, D. C. (1980). Motive dispositions: The merits of operant and respondent measures. In L. Wheeler (Ed.), *Review of personality and social psychology* (Vol. 1, pp. 10–41). Beverly Hills, CA: Sage.

McClelland, D. C. (1984a). Personal sources of my intellectual interests. In *Motives, personality, and society: Selected papers* (pp. 1–31). New York: Praeger.

McClelland, D. C. (1984b). Summary: My view of my main contributions. In *Motives, personality, and society: Selected papers* (pp. 447–466). New York: Praeger.

McClelland, D. C., & Apicella, F. S. (1945). A functional classification of verbal reactions to experimentally induced failure. *Journal of Abnormal and Social Psychology, 40,* 376–390.

McClelland, D. C., & Apicella, F. S. (1947). Reminiscence following experimentally induced failure. *Journal of Experimental Psychology, 37,* 159–169.

McClelland, D. C., & Atkinson, J. W. (1948). The projective expression of needs. I: The effect of different intensities of the hunger drive on perception. *Journal of Psychology, 25,* 205–232.

McClelland, D. C., Atkinson, J. W., & Clark, R. A. (1949). The projective expression of needs. III: The effect of ego-involvement, success, and failure on perception. *Journal of Psychology, 27,* 311–330.

McClelland, D. C., Atkinson, J. W., Clark, R. A., & Lowell, E. L. (1953). *The achievement motive.* New York: Appleton-Century-Crofts.

McClelland, D. C., Clark, R. A., Roby, T. B., & Atkinson, J. W. (1949). The projective expression of needs. IV: The effect of the need for achievement on thematic apperception. *Journal of Experimental Psychology, 39,* 242–255.

McClelland, D. C., Koestner, R., & Weinberger, J. (1989). How do self-attributed and implicit motives differ? *Psychological Review, 96,* 690–702.

McClelland, D. C., & Winter, D. G. (1969). *Motivating economic achievement.* New York: Free Press.

McKay, J. R. (1992). Affiliative trust–mistrust. In C. P. Smith (Ed.), *Motivation and personality: Handbook of thematic content analysis* (pp. 254–265). New York: Cambridge University Press.

Miller, J. G. (1939). Discrimination without awareness. *American Journal of Psychology, 52,* 562–578.

Morgan, C. D., & Murray, H. A. (1935). A method for examining fantasies: The Thematic Apperception Test. *Archives of Neurology and Psychiatry, 34,* 289–306.

Murray, H. A. (1933). The effects of fear upon estimates of the maliciousness of other personalities. *Journal of Social Psychology, 4,* 310–329.

Murray, H. A. (Ed.). (1938). *Explorations in personality: A clinical and experimental study of fifty men of college age.* New York: Oxford University Press.

Murray, H. A. (1943). *The Thematic Apperception Test: Manual.* Cambridge, MA: Harvard University Press.

Murray, H. A. (1958). Drive, time, strategy, measurement, and our way of life. In G. Lindzey (Ed.), *Assessment of human motives* (pp. 183–196). New York: Holt, Rinehart, & Winston.

Murstein, B. I. (1963). *Theory and research on projective techniques (emphasizing the TAT).* New York: Wiley.

Natti, L. M. (1946). *An investigation of certain aspects of the validity and reliability of the Thematic Apperception Test.* Unpublished master's thesis, Wesleyan University.

Robinson, F. G. (1993). *Love's story told: A life of Henry A. Murray.* Cambridge, MA: Harvard University Press.

Sanford, R. N. (1936). The effect of abstinence from food upon imaginal processes: A preliminary experiment. *Journal of Psychology, 2,* 129–136.

Sanford, R. N. (1937). The effect of abstinence from food upon imaginal processes: A further experiment. *Journal of Psychology, 3,* 145–159.

Sanford, R. N., Adkins, M. M., Miller, R. B., & Cobb, E. A. (1943). Physique, personality and scholarship. *Monographs of the Society for Research on Child Development, 8,* 1–705.

Sears, R. R. (1937). Initiation of the repression sequence by experienced failure. *Journal of Experimental Psychology, 7,* 151–163.

Shneidman, E. S. (1951). *Thematic test analysis.* New York: Grune & Stratton.

Silverman, L. H., Lachmann, F. M., & Milich, R. H. (1982). *The search for oneness.* New York: International Universities Press.

Smith, C. P. (1992a). Appendix: Pictures used to elicit thematic apperception stories. In C. P. Smith (Ed.), *Motivation and personality: Handbook of thematic content analysis* (pp. 631–647). New York: Cambridge University Press.

Smith, C. P. (Ed.). (1992b). *Motivation and personality: Handbook of thematic content analysis.* New York: Cambridge University Press.

Stein, M. I. (1955). *The Thematic Apperception Test: An introductory manual for its clinical use with adults.* Cambridge, MA: Addison-Wesley.

Stewart, A. J. (1982). The course of individual adaptation to life changes. *Journal of Personality and Social Psychology, 42,* 1100–1113.

Stewart, A. J. (1992). Self-definition and social definition: Personal styles reflected in narrative style. In C. P. Smith (Ed.), *Motivation and personality: Handbook of thematic content analysis* (pp. 481–488). New York: Cambridge University Press.

Stewart, A. J., & Healy, J. M., Jr. (1992). Assessing adaptation to life changes in terms of psychological stances toward the environment. In C. P. Smith (Ed.), *Motivation and personality: Handbook of thematic content analysis* (pp. 440–450). New York: Cambridge University Press.

Stewart, A. J., & Winter, D. G. (1974). Self-definition and social definition in women. *Journal of Personality, 42,* 238–259.

Tomkins, S. S. (1947). *The Thematic Apperception Test: The theory and technique of interpretation.* New York: Grune & Stratton.

Triplet, R. G. (1983). *Henry A. Murray and the Harvard Psychological Clinic, 1926–1938: A struggle to expand the disciplinary boundaries of psychology.* Unpublished doctoral dissertation, University of New Hampshire.

Uleman, J. S. (1966). *A new TAT measure of the need for power.* Unpublished doctoral dissertation, Harvard University.

Uleman, J. S. (1972). The need for influence: Development and validation of a measure, and comparison with the need for power. *Genetic Psychology Monographs, 85,* 157–214.

Veroff, J. (1957). Development and validation of a projective measure of power motivation. *Journal of Abnormal and Social Psychology, 54,* 1–8.

Veroff, J. (1992). Thematic apperceptive methods in survey research. In C. P. Smith (Ed.), *Motivation and personality: Handbook of thematic content analysis* (pp. 100–109). New York: Cambridge University Press.

Weinberger, J., & McClelland, D. C. (1990). Cognitive versus traditional motivational models: Irreconcilable or complementary? In E. T. Higgins & R. M. Sorrentino (Eds.), *Handbook of motivation and cognition* (Vol. 2, pp. 562–597). New York: Guilford Press.

Weinberger, J., & McLeod, C. (1989, August). *The need to belong: A psychoanalytically-based affiliative motive in the McClelland–Atkinson tradition.* Paper presented at the 97th Annual Convention of the American Psychological Association, New Orleans, LA.

Weinberger, J., & Silverman, L. H. (1990). Testability and empirical verification of psychoanalytic dynamic propositions through subliminal psychodynamic activation. *Psychoanalytic Psychology, 7,* 299–339.

Winter, D. G. (1973). *The power motive.* New York: Free Press.

Winter, D. G. (1982). David C. McClelland: An intellectual biography. In A. J. Stewart (Ed.), *Motivation and personality* (pp. xix–xxxiv). San Francisco: Jossey-Bass.

Winter, D. G. (1991). Measuring personality at a distance: Development of an integrated system for scoring motives in running text. In A. J. Stewart, J. M. Healy, Jr., & D. Ozer (Eds.), *Perspectives in personality: Approaches to understanding lives* (pp. 59–89). London: Kingsley.

Winter, D. G. (1992a). Content analysis of archival materials, personal documents, and everyday verbal productions. In C. P. Smith (Ed.), *Motivation and personality: Handbook of thematic content analysis* (pp. 110–125). New York: Cambridge University Press.

Winter, D. G. (1992b). Responsibility. In C. P. Smith (Ed.), *Motivation and personality: Handbook of thematic content analysis* (pp. 500–505). New York: Cambridge University Press.

Winter, D. G. (1993). Power, affiliation, and war: Three tests of a motivational model. *Journal of Personality and Social Psychology, 65,* 532–545.

Winter, D. G. (1996). *Personality: Analysis and interpretation of lives.* New York: McGraw-Hill.

Winter, D. G. (1998). "Toward a science of personality psychology": David McClelland's development of empirically derived TAT motive measures. *History of Psychology, 1,* 130–153.

Winter, D. G., & Barenbaum, N. B. (1985). Responsibility and the power motive in women and men. *Journal of Personality, 53,* 335–355.

Winter, D. G., & Stewart, A. J. (1977). Power motive reliability as a function of retest instructions. *Journal of Consulting and Clinical Psychology, 45,* 436–440.

10

A Personological Approach to the Thematic Apperception Test

Morris I. Stein

I am a classicist. In my Thematic Apperception Test (TAT) manual (Stein, 1948, 1955, 1981) and TAT workshops, I do everything I can to make it possible for others to share in the excitement of analyzing and interpreting a TAT protocol, as I felt when I worked with Harry Murray.

Before my graduate education was interrupted by duty in the U.S. Army during World War 2, I was Murray's research assistant at Harvard University. I attended his seminars with others who later made their marks in the TAT field, including Robert White, Silvan Tomkins, Fred Wyatt, and Robert Holt. At these seminars, we would present TAT stories and then in turn give our interpretations, which Murray noted on the blackboard. Then, came Murray's turn. It was an awesome experience. Not only did Murray integrate what everyone else had said, but he highlighted material and presented interpretations and insights that we all had missed.

I also spent hours in a little closet where Murray had deposited years and years of all kinds of magazines—for example, *Look, Life, Time*—loaded with countless photographs of all sizes from which I selected pictures for potential projective tests. There was a "mind reading test," a montage test, and others, some of which had possibilities but none of which went beyond the "experimental" stage. The noteworthy achievement of my assistantship was my research that formed part of an article that Murray published: "A Note on the Selection of Combat Officers" (Murray & Stein, 1943)." The article foreshadows Murray's future involvement in the assessment program of the Central Intelligence Agency's forerunner, the Office of Strategic Services, which I eventually joined (see Office of Strategic Services Assessment Staff, 1948). I gained intensive and extensive experience in need–press scoring of the TAT and integrated the findings into psychodynamic assessment. In this chapter, I discuss aspects of my experience with the TAT that continue to have contemporary relevance.

The Concept *Test*

Many psychologists were trained in a precise way to ask questions and the specific criteria for scoring responses. Implicitly, these psychologists are "evaluative" and essentially passive or re-active, in the sense that they use criteria developed by others. This orientation has to be overcome because it essentially leads to a "trained incapacity" to use the TAT.

In interpreting the TAT, the psychologist should not be evaluative but should aim at understanding the person who told the stories. When administering the TAT, the psychologist should try to understand the storyteller so well that he or she is capable of seeing the world as the storyteller does. The aim is to put oneself in the patient's shoes. One can check how well one is doing in this regard by listening to the first few stories and then trying to predict what the storyteller will say about pictures later in the series.

It is crucial that the TAT administrator keep in mind that he or she and the storyteller are really communicating with each other throughout the stories. For that, I find it best to think of the TAT as an "unstructured method," and my goal is to understand everything involved in the structure and content that the storyteller develops. (The word *test* implies evaluation, which the TAT should not be when administered.)

Projective Hypothesis

Tests like the Rorschach and TAT were dubbed "projective techniques" primarily as a result of Frank's (1939) article, "Projective Methods for the Study of Personality." This does not mean much now, but back then it caused some confusion. Some persisted in associating the term *projective* with the psychoanalytic concept *projection,* a defense mechanism. Although evidence might be found in the stories for projection as a defense mechanism, the dynamics behind the development of the stories were not based on it.

Frank did not intend to confuse people. He used the word *projective* in the colloquial sense of "projecting oneself" as in "projecting one's voice." In other words, in telling stories, Frank felt that the person projected his or her personality in the content and structure of the stories.[1]

Once, when I met Frank at the Harvard Psychological Clinic, I teased him about the confusion he caused. He responded by saying that he always felt his article on projective techniques should be regarded as a railroad timetable—good until a certain time but not beyond. I could not agree more. It is interesting that the designation of projective techniques has persisted to this day, but the confusion has faded.

I have always preferred using the words *unstructured tests* or *unstructured methods.* I teach that the psychologist's task is to make sense out of how and why the participant structures the stories the way he or she does.

---

[1]In *Explorations in Personality,* Murray (1938) referred to the TAT and other methods to uncover conscious material as "projection tests," using this term as similar to Frank's "projective techniques."

Clinician's Intuition

Interpreting a TAT is often described as an art, not a science, and good interpreters are sometimes described as intuitive. Some psychologists love these designations; others are indifferent. Still others say they have no intuition and are not artists and, therefore, shy away from the TAT. In the face of a TAT protocol, these psychologists are intimidated and almost catatonic. I attempt to counteract these effects.

In my published interpretations and teaching of the TAT, I try my best to provide the psychological rationale for any statement I make and frequently in a great deal of detail. No use is made of such statements as "it feels like this or that." The purpose is to verbalize, as best I can, the reason for each analytic and interpretative statement.

If someone argues that the whole interpretative process is based on psychoanalytic theory or another theory, I do not argue but engage the person in the use of whatever personality theory they desire to apply to TAT interpretations. This is usually effective in winning people over to work with the TAT.

Some TAT teachers and interpreters find it worthwhile to use theoretical jargon—the language of "object relationships," of Sigmund Freud, Carl Jung, or Heinz Kohut, and so forth—but in my work, I avoid technical jargon to best help neophytes feel comfortable.

Value of Murray's Needs and Press

Although I focus on demonstrating to students that they can use the knowledge they already have to interpret the TAT, I believe it is worthwhile to try to score the TAT in terms of Murray's "needs" and "press." Murray's system is foreign to most psychologists, and its neologisms may be particularly frustrating. But it is a good exercise to score at least a few TATs in this way because it forces the interpreter to concentrate on every word in the stories. The detailed definitions of Murray's variables and the distinctions between them can alert the psychologist to significant data that would otherwise be overlooked. I find that a periodic reading of the sections on needs and press in *Explorations in Personality* (Murray, 1938) is invaluable to turning up the "third ear" that is sensitized to psychodynamic phenomena.

Number of Cards to Use

For clinical diagnostic purposes, I have used Murray's recommended set of 20 adult TAT cards as part of a test battery administered in two sessions. But as the occasion demands—usually for executive selection—I have used fewer cards that have been either selected from the Murray cards or developed by an industrial consultant for specific purposes. I feel quite comfortable with various sets of cards and encourage students to be flexible and to learn about different sets, so that they will be able to deal with the diversity of assessment tasks that may confront them.

Administration

For clinical and selection purposes, one has to be ready to adapt to the situation and to vary the procedure for recording stories. Having used a variety of techniques, I still prefer writing the stories as the storyteller tells them to me. I feel closer to the storyteller and more sensitive to nuances in behavior, voice quality, and interactions that I might otherwise miss. There are times, however, when this is not possible, and I have made do with handwritten or recorded stories.

Test Battery

The TAT is best used as part of a test battery whether for clinical diagnostic purposes or selection purposes. In most instances, depending on the needs of the case, I prefer starting with an interview. This is followed by an intelligence test, or a measure of cognitive functioning, and the first part of the Stein Sentence Completion Test (SSCT; Stein, 1947, 1949).[2] I then administer the first 10 cards of the regular TAT. This is followed by the second part of the SSCT on the assumption that it will elicit material that has been "stirred up" by the TAT. This completes the first session. The second session starts with an interview, followed by the Rorschach Test, the second half of the regular TAT set, and a concluding interview.

Information About Levels of Personality

The test battery just described makes it possible to make a statement about the level at which some material might appear or be. Is the behavior manifest or latent? Is it conscious or unconscious? Or under what conditions might it occur? Such determinations should be made by the psychologist albeit very carefully and cautiously. As a description, I regard the Rorschach as the skeleton of the personality, the TAT the flesh around it, and the SSCT the skin. The SSCT is most likely to provide data at the most manifest and conscious levels—that which the storyteller is most aware of—and the Rorschach and the TAT provide information at the "deeper" levels.

---

[2]The SSCT consists of 100 items in two sets of 50 items each. "Personal" and "third person" sentence stems are presented in an attempt to elicit material both directly and indirectly (projectively). The SSCT was designed to gather information in the following areas: family, past, drives, inner states, *cathexes* (investments of mental or emotional energy in a person, object, or idea), energy, time perspective, and reactions of others.

Anabolic and Catabolic Characteristics

Murray used the physiology of metabolism as a metaphor to call attention to the fact that in the study of personality, it is important not only to deal with the *catabolic* characteristics (those that lead to regression and the breakdown of personality) but also to deal with the *anabolic* characteristics (those that lead to psychological development and growth). A more common way of thinking about this is to look at both the strengths and weaknesses of a person. Murray's basic point is that most psychologists look at weaknesses, not strengths, that is, catabolic, not anabolic, characteristics. A complete study of the person and the report should state both.

To facilitate thinking about these matters, I presented in my manual (Stein, 1981) stories told for Card 17 (a man on a rope) by five different people: a successful professional man, a student with obsessive thoughts, a compulsive patient, a schizophrenia patient before and after insulin shock and psychotherapy, and a deteriorated organic patient. By focusing on how the language these people used affected their thought process as well as the content of the stories and their integration, I demonstrated how one develops sensitivity to both anabolic and catabolic characteristics of personality.

Reporting Thematic Apperception Test Findings for Selection Purposes

When using a TAT for personnel selection purposes, the client is usually interested in, among other things, the storyteller's possible social interaction with various people in an organization. To satisfy these needs, the psychologist must study the stories in an effort to determine how the storyteller may interact with three different groups of people on the job, namely, superiors, colleagues, and subordinates. If the pictures have been properly selected, the stories may well contain material directly related to interactions with these different social groups. Where this is not so, it is necessary to keep the psychodynamics of the person in mind and ask oneself how the storyteller would interact with the three different groups.

Psychologist's Role

The psychologist's role in administering, analyzing, interpreting, and integrating TAT data is most crucial. With the proper psychological stance, one feels as if one is a discoverer in an uncharted land, a participant in a mystery, a detective on a case, or a sculptor trying to discover the person within as well as the function of the external armor. One feels all these things and more because one has to draw on all that one knows about human behavior.

In analyzing and interpreting a TAT, one must not only identify the hero–heroine but also assume that what the hero–heroine says or does is true of the storyteller. To get all that a TAT protocol contains, one needs to listen with one's third ear and get the meaning behind the story. To be sure, the interpreter needs to be versed and trained in psychodynamics, but he or she also needs to be a psycholinguist, aware of cognitive factors, the dynamics of perception, and thought processes and problem solving.

When one is interpreting and integrating TAT data, hypotheses come to mind one minute, only to be clarified or rejected the next. Hopefully, new ones come to the forefront, although sometimes there are lacunae, paradoxes, and gaps. All this has to be worked through.

Next, one needs to complete the final integration for composing a psychological profile, but it is not always clear where to start. One is more like the abstract painter or the impressionist rather than the portrait painter. Somehow knowledge of personality theory and experience with TATs guides one to the final picture. A follow-up of cases and selections gives the psychologist important feedback about accuracy and error and is indispensable to the learning process.

Conclusion

According to Murray (1967), the TAT was designed to "educe (draw forth) words, sentences, or stories as ground for verifiable or plausible inferences in regard to influential components of personality which the subject is either unable or unwilling to report" (p. 304). The TAT does this and more; it also provides information about components of the personality that the participant is willing and able to report.[3]

In working with the TAT, the psychologist has to make use of his or her total experience as a psychologist. Everything one learned in psychology, including all of cognitive psychology, psychodynamic theories of personality, social psychology, linguistics, cultural anthropology, and so forth, contribute to work with the TAT. One never feels more like a psychologist than when one works with the TAT.

References

Dana, R. H. (1996). Thematic Apperception Test (TAT). In C. S. Newmark (Ed.), *Major psychological assessment instruments* (2nd ed., pp. 166–205). Needham Heights, MA: Allyn & Bacon.

Frank, L. K. (1939). Projective methods for the study of personality. *Journal of Psychology, 8,* 389–413.

Groth-Marnat, G. (1997). *Handbook of psychological assessment* (3rd ed.). New York: Wiley.

Murray, H. A. (Ed.). (1938). *Explorations in personality: A clinical and experimental study of fifty men of college age.* New York: Oxford University Press.

---

[3]Groth-Marnat (1997) discussed the typical themes elicited by each TAT card by summarizing and integrating the work of Murray, Bellak, and myself. The TAT's capacity for investigating various personality components is well illustrated. Dana (1996) also discussed typical TAT themes.

Murray, H. A. (1967). The case of Murr. In E. G. Boring & G. A. Lindzey (Eds.), *A history of psychology in autobiography* (Vol. 5, pp. 283–310). New York: Appleton-Century-Crofts.

Murray, H. A., & Stein, M. I. (1943). Note on the selection of combat officers. *Psychosomatic Medicine, 5,* 386–391.

Office of Strategic Services Assessment Staff. (1948). *Assessment of men.* New York: Rinehart.

Stein, M. I. (1947). The use of a sentence completion test for the diagnosis of personality. *Journal of Clinical Psychology, 36,* 311–322.

Stein, M. I. (1948). *The Thematic Apperception Test: A manual for its clinical use with males.* Cambridge, MA: Addison-Wesley.

Stein, M. I. (1949). The record and a sentence completion test. *Journal of Consulting Psychology, 13,* 448–449.

Stein, M. I. (1955). *The Thematic Apperception Test: A manual for its clinical use with adults* (rev. ed.) Cambridge, MA: Addison-Wesley.

Stein, M. I. (1981). *The Thematic Apperception Test: A manual for its clinical use with adults* (2nd ed.). Springfield, IL: Charles C Thomas. (Available from Mews Press, Box 2052, Amagansett, NY 11930)

11

My Perceptions of the Thematic Apperception Test in Psychodiagnosis and Psychotherapy

Leopold Bellak

I have very often been told, by colleagues and patients, that the Thematic Apperception Test (TAT) pictures are cheerless, outdated looking, and artistically undistinguished—and I agree. But they have prevailed, despite several attempts to compete with them. They seem to have a unique ability to stimulate rich and useful responses. To put it in the form of an old saw, if I were on an island and could have the choice of one single diagnostic device only, I would want it to be TAT Card 1, the picture of the youthful Yehudi Menuhin behind a violin. If in response to Card 1, someone told me that "the boy thinks about smashing the violin" and kept up that sort of theme with card after card, I would make the *observation-near inference* that this person is preoccupied with aggression. If that person was the model of a choirboy in manifest behavior, I may have a clinically important datum: This person suppresses a good deal of anger. If one is a careful clinician, one goes on cautiously to increasingly more complex, more observation-distant diagnostic inferences.

Some satisfaction with the apperceptive techniques derives then, I believe, from the fact that nothing gets between the psychologist and the patient. The TAT and the Rorschach share a source of satisfaction for the diagnostician, that is, the "aha" experience of seeing things hang together—fulfilling a need to understand things, probably a basic motivation for all clinicians.

Many psychologists are unsure as to the value of the TAT in diagnostic assessment. Their practices are characterized by inadequate methods of administration that elicit only sparse descriptions of TAT cards. Some clinicians have inconsistently chosen different cards for different test takers on the basis of which cards "pull" for which material that might resemble each test taker's personality. Interpretation of the stories is frequently based only on an impressionistic summary of themes.

I developed a scientifically consistent approach to the TAT. It entails a standard method of administration, a standard TAT sequence of 10 cards (1, 2, 3 BM, 4, 5 BM, 7 GF, 8 BM, 9 GF, 10, and 13 MF, which can be supplemented by cards that pull for specific material), and a standard method of scoring. Scoring includes Murray's (1943) scoring approach along with a more comprehensive and practical scoring system (Bellak & Abrams, 1997). This system improves the psychologist's ability to use the TAT in making clinical diagnoses and facilitating the psychotherapeutic process.

An important development in thematic testing is a multidimensional assessment approach, which is part of the Bellak scoring system. Originally, thematic tests were considered only personality tests; today, the contemporary psychologist can use an entire group of tests in the psychological test battery to evaluate all the different dimensions of cognitive–intellectual functioning, neuropsychological or learning disability assessment, creative thinking, and social–emotional functioning. Intelligence tests are no longer considered only cognitive–intellectual measures. The Bender Gestalt Test is no longer considered only a neuropsychological screening instrument, and the TAT and the Rorschach are no longer used only as projective personality tests.

Psychologists use intelligence tests to evaluate intellectual functioning; however, test behavior and other aspects of the intelligence test also reveal many aspects of the test taker's personality. The Bender Gestalt Test is primarily used for screening perceptual–motor neuropsychological functioning; however, specific evaluation of line pressure, spacing of designs, and size of designs also reveal a lot about the test taker's personality characteristics. Thematic tests are primarily windows into the inner feelings, conflicts, defense and coping mechanisms, interpersonal relations, and other personality factors of the test taker. Psychologists also use these tests to obtain a sample of language usage, evaluate the level of logical thinking in the organization of story elements into a coherent whole, and evaluate other aspects of cognitive, intellectual, and neuropsychological functioning of the test taker (see Bellak & Abrams, 1997, for two examples of using the TAT in cases of attention deficit disorder).

Nearer to the area of my own competence is the ever-increasing role of brief psychotherapy and the important contributions apperceptive techniques can make to that field (Bellak, Abrams, & Ackerman-Engel, 1992). Brief therapy, after all, is only possible if one can make a concise psychodiagnosis to have a clear conceptualization as a guide for concise interventions.

Similarly, liaison psychiatrists can use psychodiagnosis through apperceptive techniques, not only for diagnostic labels but also as a focus for treatment. If one has a great deal of preoperative anxiety or postoperative depression, one's TAT stories may provide rich insight into the dynamic meaning of the malady for this particular person. In the case of psychosomatic disorder, recent work shows that the TAT may also be very useful in illuminating the related psychodynamic features. The TAT can unify again the role of clinician as diagnostician and therapist.

Psychodiagnosis

In 1944, I was still struggling experimentally with the mystique of projection myself. At first, I resolved the problem by speaking of adaptive, expressive, and projective aspects of responses to tests (Bellak, 1944). Next, I brought ego psychology to bear on the response by studying defenses in the TAT and then changed from speaking of projection to apperceptive distortion (Bellak, 1950a, 1950b, 1954). Eventually, I found Kris's (1950, 1952) concept of adaptive regression in the service of the ego perhaps most useful for understanding the creative process involved in responses. Adaptive regression in the service of the ego can be translated as a brief, oscillating, relative reduction of certain adaptive functions of the ego in the service of other, specifically the "synthetic," ego functions. Cognitive, selective, adaptive functions are then decreased. This weakens the sharply defined boundaries of figure and ground of logical, temporal, spatial, and other relations; permits unconscious material to become conscious; and leads to a reordering into new configurations with new boundaries under the scrutiny of the again sharply functioning adaptive forces (Bellak, 1993).

My increasing knowledge and understanding of ego pathology helped me in relating manifest content and latent content revealed in testing. As I considered ego functions as intervening variables, the richest yield came from understanding the value of the discrepancy of what goes on relatively latently and what is manifest: Discrepancy helps in assessing the forces of control and of cognition and aids in the prediction of clinical course.

On the broader scene, the interaction between laboratory psychology and clinical psychology similarly comes to embrace responses to projective tests as individual differences in perception effected by interlocking motivations. What I tried to describe as expressive aspects has since been highly developed into the field of cognitive style. Interplay among adaptive functions of the ego, environment, and drive has become a staple of psychological science, from motivational research to clinical and social psychology (see McClelland, chap. 13; and Winter, chap. 9, this volume).

Projective methods as diagnostic devices are, then, much less of a theoretical problem today than they were in the past and, by that token, much less of a methodological problem (Bellak, 1992). If one desires to computerize projective test responses, one only has to work out good definitions of terms for use in content analytic studies (on the basis of frequency of word order, narrative action sequence, and other objective scoring variables) to make these techniques acceptable to the hardest of psychological hardware specialists.

A diagnostic concept, it should be noted, is a heuristic hypothesis. It should involve propositions concerning the etiology, treatment, and prognosis of the disease or syndrome under consideration. The diagnostic hypothesis must be measured by the traditional scientific criteria of validity and reliability. In the broadest sense, the usefulness of a diagnostic hypothesis is indicated by its ability to help one understand, predict, and control. To understand means to see how the particular set of conditions involved in the diagnosis fit into the matrix of a sequence of causal events.

It is in this significance that I speak of psychodynamic diagnosis: relating the patient one meets to the biosociopsychological facts of his or her life and trying to understand the relationship of his or her drives, ego and superego controls, value systems, and adaptive problems to the complaints that bring him or her to the psychologist.

To have maximal usefulness, a diagnosis must have nomothetic and idiographic aspects. There must be enough of general propositions to see the symptoms of a person as roughly belonging to a class of disorder—for example, neurosis and psychosis, specifically what kind of neurosis, psychosis, or other class of maladaptive functioning—so that one may make general inferences with regard to prediction (prognosis) and treatment. Within the nomothetic group a person belongs to, there is also concern with the idiographic features, the identification of those factors that make the person uniquely himself or herself above and beyond group membership.

The nomothetic diagnosis implies that psychologists deal with at least a quasistable characteristic: a gestalt of drives, controls, and environmental input that has enough discreteness to assure more intragroup similarity between people in the given nosological group than intergroup similarity. It also implies that this characteristic constellation has a stable enough temporal quality to be usefully so identified. However, by virtue of thinking in dynamic terms, it must also be obvious and stated that a person has more or less of a propensity to move toward other forms of compromise formation between the different forces. Not only must a diagnosis, then, establish nosological class properties that are useful for cataloging a person for statistical purposes and about which a general statement can be made, but it must also state the unique properties at the time of diagnosis and the individual likelihood of continuing or moving, for better or for worse, to another form of adaptiveness—healthier, sicker, or just different qualitatively (Bellak, 1993).

Psychotherapy

The TAT is particularly valuable as a vehicle of the psychotherapeutic process in cases where therapy of necessity must be short term or in emergency situations (self-endangering or extremely crippling depressions or acute anxiety). As first proposed by Morgan and Murray (1935), the TAT is recommended for brief psychotherapy because it may quickly reveal situational and psychodynamic issues that need discussing. One may select those pictures that are most apt to bring out the problems of a specific patient where time is of the essence for external or internal reasons (Bellak et al., 1992). For example, stories for Card 3 GF (a woman standing with her head downcast and her face covered with her hands) or Card 14 (the silhouette of a man or woman against a bright window) may be helpful for a patient who is severely depressed or suicidal.

Cooperation and insight for both therapist and patient are frequently gained when patients discover, to their surprise, in their TAT stories that they have unwittingly reproduced some of their most important problems. The TAT may be especially useful when the patient has severe difficulty in communicating because of a lack of familiarity with the psychotherapeutic process, inhibitions, or resistance.

Patients not used to any degree of objective introspection consider their complaints to be purely organic or environmentally caused. Very often when denial interferes with communication and insight, reading back several stories may dramatically bring home to the patient the operation of denial. Two cards, especially Card 2 (one character appears to be pregnant) and Card 3 BM (a figure huddled by a couch with a gun on the floor), have been useful in such situations; with these cards, it is relatively easy to show the patient how denial has caused them to exclude from their perception objects and circumstances of such visibility. The operation of denial may then be interpreted in specific aspects of the patient's own real-life behavior with greater insight than would otherwise be forthcoming.

One very important use of the TAT is to help some patients gain necessary "distance" from themselves and to develop a psychotherapeutic attitude. Adolescents pressured by their parents to go to therapy but not openly hostile may present with an isolation of affect and intellectualization, denying any emotional problems or troubling feelings. After creating even brief TAT stories, they can be asked what they think of the stories. The initial response frequently is that the stories are about pictures that have nothing to do with them. The first step, then, is for the therapist to tell the patient that he or she has heard many different stories about these pictures and that the patient's stories differ from others' stories. As an illustration, the patient can be given examples of themes different from those in the patient's stories. This fact of being different often makes a strong impression, supplying the therapist with an entering wedge.

The therapist and patient can now consider why the patient's stories are the way they are rather than like other people's stories. For instance, a defensive male adolescent may tell stories that actually show a great deal of despair and anxiety that is nevertheless denied. The therapist may then read someone else's less disturbed stories and ask the adolescent what the difference is between his stories and the others'. Insight may slowly emerge, and he may admit that his stories show some unhappiness. The therapist may ask why and, if necessary, point out specific circumstances of unhappiness in the stories, such as loneliness, fear of failure, and feelings of inadequacy.

A preferable approach, in less defensive cases, is to hand the patient several of his or her own stories and ask him or her to play psychologist and tell the therapist what the stories have in common. This way, the patient may learn to look for patterns in his or her behavior and emotions, and the process of "working through" or resolution may start. Sometimes a central problem otherwise unapproachable except in long-term therapy can be broached in this way.

The TAT is capable of revealing cognitions, fantasies, and psychodynamics that even a skilled psychotherapist may not anticipate or discern after several therapy sessions. In ongoing psychotherapy, it is advisable to introduce the TAT if the patient does not present any acute problems, has difficulty starting, or quickly runs out of material during sessions. As the therapist interprets the TAT in such cases, the patient should be encouraged to bring up more distantly related emotional issues that were evoked and to discuss current problems that could not be verbalized before. This procedure often has the effect of increasing the patient's awareness, especially of preconscious thoughts and feelings. Therapy can then proceed according to the patterns revealed in the TAT stories and the associations the patient makes to them.

The ways in which the TAT may be used in individual therapy are further discussed elsewhere by myself and others (Bellak & Abrams, 1997; Bellak, Pasquarelli, & Braverman, 1949; Hermans, chap. 16, this volume; Hoffman & Kuperman, 1990; Holzbert, 1963; Meyer & Tolman, 1955; Peterson, 1990; Rosenzweig, chap. 4, this volume). Araoz (1972) showed how it is useful in couples therapy. Given its focus on interpersonal relationships, the TAT can be helpful in selecting group therapy candidates (Ullman, 1957) and can be jointly interpreted by psychotherapists and patients as part of group therapy itself (Hoffman, Rosner, Danon, & Peres, 1993).

Psychoanalysis and Perception

Personality assessment, using the TAT, Children's Apperception Test, and Senior Apperception Test (Bellak & Abrams, 1997), among other means, is a method of studying individual perceptual differences and of understanding them as the unique product of the interaction of personal history with external and organismic factors in the present, in the past, and at different points in the future. Psychoanalysis, the theoretical bedrock of such assessment, was always, among other things, a perceptual theory. When it is not busy being a theory of motivation; developmental theory; broadly speaking, learning theory; dynamic theory of interacting forces; or systems theory, as in psychosomatic medicine; psychoanalysis is concerned with the effect of earlier perceptions on contemporary perceptions.

In apperceptive techniques, individual differences in perceptual distortion of standard stimuli are studied. By looking for interpersonal common denominators as well as interpersonal differences, psychologists hope to glimpse the unique perceptions of an individual and one's ways of coping with what is perceived. It is as simple as all that. Quantitative content analysis is still not used enough to put these inferences on a statistically respectable basis. One would think some bright young computer specialist would program his or her gadgets to not only count words but also analyze clusters of what Murray called syndromes of *press* and *need*—units of stimulus and drive. These clusters should give a lively picture of a personality and keep methodologists happy.

Sigmund Freud's basic contribution to the field of personality theory and perceptions was to establish continuity between childhood and adulthood, between waking thought and dreaming thought, and between "normality" and psychopathology. He established causality in psychological science. This is his unique contribution, unprecedented, unparalleled, and unsurpassed. Apperceptive, projective techniques are predicated on these basic hypotheses. The specific responses to the stimuli are determined by specific factors. One need not use the narrowest kind of mechanistic determinism to maintain these propositions. A high degree of probability of relationships is a very adequate basis for psychologists' work.

Personality Theory

Personality theory holds that personality is a relatively stable system. For example, one expects Tom Jones to be approximately the same person today, tomorrow, and the next year as he was yesterday and 1 month ago. However, of course, one knows that a patient may have been depressed yesterday and be anxious tomorrow and that successively administered tests, like the TAT, would reflect these changes and still reveal the basic structure.

In interpreting apperceptive responses, the psychologist must know something about the participant's current life situation. One wants to make sure that the participant does not have a temperature of 103° when taking the test. But with all other things being equal, psychologists are betting that the main personality organization is being reliably and validly revealed. It is most useful to see the participant's responses to stimuli and to the instructions as a task with which the participant has to cope. Personality, symptomatology, and style are then best studied as copying mechanisms. Their adequacy, usefulness, or pathology are the broadest basis for diagnostic inferences.

Within the last 2 decades, object relations theory has attracted a good deal of interest. In terms of the discussions so far, this simply means that certain perceptual aspects, namely, the precepts concerned with self-representation as well as the interaction of internalized object relations, have received more attention than they have previously. Object relations theory simply emphasizes, in various forms by different authors, the specific effect of self-perceptions at different times of one's development and of object perceptions at different stages on contemporary perception. To use Henry Murray's term, self- and object representations have a "regnant" effect on perception.

This perspective is very useful in studying responses to the TAT and is not in conflict with basic psychoanalytic theory or the way I have always interpreted responses to these stimuli. Those who like Kohut's (1971, 1974) contributions to self-psychology may find it useful to read a case study that my colleague Abrams (1993) illustrated with a thematic test protocol of narcissistic pathology. I believe that the field of TAT assessment needs more such clinical case protocols, which include multiple diagnostic perspectives from different schools of psychotherapy. This line of study could facilitate a shared understanding of the clinical use of thematic tests.

Conclusion

In planning a patient's treatment, a psychologist must obtain as much advance information as possible. The TAT and other apperceptive techniques meet this need. Apperceptive techniques provide data that are useful for understanding virtually any facet of the human mind and can be used therapeutically.

The stories people tell are primary documents. They are the unique products of the storyteller. By what criteria an investigator wants to study the uniqueness of each production is the investigator's choice. In that sense, the TAT is a monument to humanism. To paraphrase what Freud said of the dream, I provide this description: It is a royal road to the understanding of the individual and thus to all of the human spectacle. Therefore, the TAT and related techniques are likely to remain part of the psychological and psychiatric fields, come what may.

References

Abrams, D. M. (1993). Pathological narcissism in an eight-year-old boy: An example of Bellak's T.A.T. and C.A.T. diagnostic system. *Psychoanalytic Psychology, 10,* 573–591.

Araoz, D. L. (1972). The Thematic Apperception Test in marital therapy. *Journal of Contemporary Psychotherapy, 5,* 41–48.

Bellak, L. (1944). The concept of projection: An experimental investigation and study of the concept. *Psychiatry, 7,* 353–370.

Bellak, L. (1950a). On the problems of the concept of projection. In L. Abt & L. Bellak (Eds.), *Projective psychology* (pp. 7–33). New York: Knopf.

Bellak, L. (1950b). Thematic apperception: Failures and the defenses. *Transactions of the New York Academy of Science* [Series 2], *12,* 112–126.

Bellak, L. (1954). *The T.A.T. and C.A.T. in clinical use.* New York: Grune & Stratton.

Bellak, L. (1992). Projective techniques in the computer age (Bruno Klopfer Award). *Journal of Personality Assessment, 58,* 445–453.

Bellak, L. (1993). *Psychoanalysis as a science.* Boston: Allyn & Bacon.

Bellak, L., & Abrams, D. M. (1997). *The T.A.T., the C.A.T. and the S.A.T. in clinical use* (6th ed.). Needham Heights, MA: Allyn & Bacon.

Bellak, L., Abrams, D. M., & Ackerman-Engel, R. (1992). *Handbook of intensive brief and emergency psychotherapy.* Larchmont, NY: CPS.

Bellak, L., Pasquarelli, B., & Braverman, S. (1949). The use of the Thematic Apperception Test in psychotherapy. *Journal of Nervous and Mental Disease, 110,* 51–65.

Hoffman, S., & Kuperman, N. (1990). Indirect treatment of traumatic psychological experiences: The use of the TAT cards. *American Journal of Psychotherapy, 44,* 107–115.

Hoffman, S., Rosner, L., Danon, A., & Peres, R. (1993). Use of the TAT in group therapy with children. *Journal of Child and Adolescent Group Therapy, 3,* 121–128.

Holzbert, J. (1963). Projective techniques and resistance to change in psychotherapy as viewed through a communications model. *Journal of Projective Techniques, 27,* 430–435.

Kohut, H. (1971). *The analysis of the self.* New York: International Universities Press.

Kohut, H. (1974). *Restoration of the self.* Middleton, CT: International Universities Press.

Kris, E. (1950). On preconscious mental processes. *Psychoanalytic Quarterly, 19,* 540–560.

Kris, E. (1952). *Psychoanalytic explorations of art.* New York: International Universities Press.

Meyer, M. M., & Tolman, R. S. (1955). Parental figures in Sentence Completion Test, in T.A.T., and in therapeutic interviews. *Journal of Consulting Psychology, 19,* 170.

Morgan, C. D., & Murray, H. A. (1935). A method for investigating fantasies: The Thematic Apperception Test. *Archives of Neurological Psychiatry, 34,* 289–306.

Murray, H. A. (1943). *Thematic Apperception Test: Manual.* Cambridge, MA: Harvard University Press.

Peterson, C. A. (1990). Administration of the Thematic Apperception Test: Contributions of psychoanalytic psychotherapy. *Journal of Contemporary Psychotherapy, 20,* 191–200.

Ullman, L. (1957). Selection of neuropsychiatric patients for group psychotherapy. *Journal of Consulting Psychology, 21,* 277–280.

12

Six Decades of the Bellak Scoring System, Among Others

David M. Abrams

In this chapter, I describe Leopold Bellak's contributions to the clinical utility of the Thematic Apperception Test (TAT). Personality research by Bellak and other TAT proponents is reviewed. The theoretical and practical multidimensionality of the TAT is discussed, and recommendations for further development are provided.

Bellak Enters the Thematic Apperception Test Picture

Bellak was born in Vienna, Austria, was a childhood friend of one of Sigmund Freud's grandchildren (the child psychoanalyst Ernst Freud), and began his psychoanalytic training during his years at the University of Vienna. When Hitler invaded Vienna in 1938, Bellak immigrated to the United States where he enrolled in the New York Medical College. Shortly thereafter, he interrupted medical school to study for a couple of years with Harry Murray at Harvard University and obtained a master's in psychology.

Bellak and Murray remained close friends until Murray's death at the age of 95. Bellak once saved Murray's life by flying to where the Murrays were vacationing when he heard that Murray was ill (Nina Murray, personal communication, April 1998).

One of the very first scoring schemes for the TAT was by Murray and Bellak (1941; also see Bellak, 1950b). As Table 12.1 illustrates, 35 "needs" are listed in one column and 32 "presses" listed in another. The form includes a checklist for individuals mentioned in each story, whether they were "allies" of, or "opposing," the main hero–heroine.

Murray welcomed Bellak's perspective on the TAT, which was influenced by S. Freud's (1923) later theory of ego psychology. Although Murray was interested in psychoanalysis, he was more critical of Freud than Bellak, especially in light of his Jungian sentiments. The reader may find it historically interesting that Bellak managed to persuade Murray to include the two Freudian drives of sexuality and aggression in this early scoring approach. However, by the time of Murray's (1943) publication of

Table 12.1. Murray and Bellak's Interpretation Categories for the Thematic Apperception Test

Picture No.				Quantitative data			
Needs	n	Of	Weight score	Press	p	Op	Weight score
Abasement: Submission Intragg: Verbal				*Personal* Acquisition: Social			
Physical				Asocial			
Achievement				Affiliation: Associative			
Acquisition: Social				Emotional			
Asocial				Aggression: Verbal			
Affiliation: Associative				Physical: Social			
Emotional				Asocial			
Aggression: Verbal				Curiosity			
Physical: Social				Deference: Compliance			
Asocial				Respect			
Destruction				Dominance: Coercion			
Autonomy: Freedom				Restraint			
Negativism				Exposition			
Asocial				Gratuity			
Blame avoidance				Nurturance			
Change				Punishment			
Cognizance				Rejection			
Counteraction				Retention			
Deference: Compliance				Sex			
Respect				Succorance			
Dominance				*Impersonal*			
Excitance				Affliction: Mental			
Exhibition				Physical			
Harm avoidance				Claustrum			
Infavoidance				Death			
Nurturance				Imposed task			
Nutriance				Insupport			
Organization				Physical danger: Active			
Passivity				Insupport			
Playmirth				Physical injury			
Recognition				Lack			
Rejection				Loss			

(Table continues)

Table 12.1. (*Continued*)

Picture No.				Quantitative data			
Retention				Luck: Good			
Seclusion				Bad			
Sentience: Epicurean				Monotony			
Aesthetic							
Sex				Failure			
Succorance				Accomplishment			

	Allied		Opposing	
People	M	F	M	F
Superior				
Parent				
Government				
Equal				
Sibling				
Spouse				
Lover				
Group				
Inferior				
Offspring				

Note. F = female; Intragg = intraggression; M = male; n = need; p = press; Of = allies of the hero; Op = opposing the hero. From *Thematic Apperception Test Blank* [unpublished mimeograph], by H. A. Murray and L. Bellak, 1941, Cambridge, MA: Harvard Psychological Clinic. Copyright 1941 by Leopold Bellak, MD. Reprinted with permission.

the TAT and the TAT manual, the sexual or pleasure need was dropped, whereas aggression was retained in the scoring system.

Murray's final system in the TAT manual includes the needs of abasement, achievement, aggression, acquisition, autonomy, creation, deference, destruction, dominance, intraggression, nurturance, passivity, succorance, and a list of forces that press on the individual and often oppose the individual's needs of affiliation, aggression, dominance, nurturance, lack, loss, or physical injury. Murray believed that this dualistic need–press approach provides a way to assess an individual's relationship to the environment. Murray also felt that there are patterns of need–press relationships in each individual personality, which the series of TAT stories can reveal.

Bellak (1944) conducted one of the first experimental studies using the TAT in an examination of the defense mechanism of projection. This would have been his PhD dissertation were it not for Murray's insistence that Bellak would do better to return to New York Medical College and first complete his MD. However, he did finally publish this experiment, which was replicated many years later by Phebe Cramer (1991a). Cramer (1996) also incorporated part of Bellak's (1950a, 1950b, 1950c, 1950d) way of scoring projection on the TAT by scoring the introduction of figures, objects, and events that are not in the picture.

Bellak's Thematic Apperception Test Scoring System

Bellak (1955; personal communication, May 1999) orginally called his scoring system the "Bellak TAT short form." It includes 10 categories of analysis that are spread out on a 3-page scoring form. The 10 categories are outlined on the left column of the first page, and each of the 10 TAT stories can be scored according to these 10 categories, along vertical columns from left-to-right to the third page, one column for each TAT story.

Bellak was influenced by the multidimensional approach of Sigmund Freud's (1923) metapsychological assumptions and structural or ego psychology theory and Anna Freud's (e.g., 1965) developmental or diagnostic profile as well as the multidimensional categories used in the clinical mental status evaluation. The mental status evaluation assesses a patient's functioning in the following areas: emotions and mood; appropriateness of affect; defense organization; organization or looseness of fantasy; degree of reality testing; degree of thinking; orientation to person, place, and time; and degree of perceptual functioning. In his TAT scoring system, Bellak's 10 categories include the following (see Table 12.2):

1. Main theme
2. Identity and functioning of the main hero (male, female, competent, ineffectual)
3. Main needs of the hero (the heritage from Murray's scoring of needs)
4. Conception of the world (heritage from Murray's environmental press)
5. Interpersonal object relations (main hero's relation to peers and senior and junior figures)
6. Significant conflicts
7. Nature of fears, insecurities, and anxieties
8. Main defense and coping mechanisms
9. Moral or superego functioning
10. Integration of the ego (seen in story outcome, formal story characteristics, and other ego functions).

Table 12.2. Bellak's TAT Short Form

	Story no. 1	Story no. 2
1. Main theme: (diagnostic level; if descriptive and interpretative levels are desired, use a scratch sheet)		
2. Main hero–heroine: age _____ sex _____ vocation _____ abilities _____ interests _____ traits _____ body image _____ adequacy _____ self-image _____		
3. Main needs and drives of hero–heroine (a) behavioral needs (as in story) _____ implying _____ (b) figure, objects, or circumstances introduced _____ implying need for or to _____ (c) figures, objects, or circumstances omitted _____ implying need for or to _____		
4. Conception of environment (world) as _____		
5. (a) Parental figures (m ___, f ___) are seen as _____ and participant's reaction to a is _____ (b) Contemporary figures (m ___, f ___) are seen as _____ and participant's reaction to b is _____ (c) Junior figures (m ___, f ___) are seen as _____ and participant's reaction to c is _____		
6. Significant conflicts _____		
7. Nature of anxieties of physical harm or punishment _____ of disapproval _____ of lack or loss of love _____ of illness or injury _____ of being deserted _____ of deprivation _____ of being overpowered and helpless _____ of being devoured _____ other _____		
8. Main defenses against conflicts and fears repression _____ reaction–formation _____ regression _____ denial _____ introjection _____ isolation _____ undoing _____ rationalization _____ other _____		
9. Adequacy of superego as manifested by "punishment" for "crime" being appropriate _____ inappropriate _____ too severe (also indicated by immediacy of punishment) _____ inconsistent _____ too lenient _____ also _____		

(Table continues)

Table 12.2. *(Continued)*

delayed initial response or pauses _____		
stammer _____ other manifestations of		
superego interference _____		
10. Integration of the ego, manifesting itself in		
hero: adequate _____ inadequate _____		
outcome: happy _____ unhappy _____	- - - - -	- - - - -
realistic _____ unrealistic _____		
drive control _____	- - - - -	- - - - -
thought processes as revealed by plot being		
stereotyped _____ original _____ appropriate _____		
complete _____ incomplete _____ inappropriate _____		
syncretic _____ concrete _____ contaminated _____	- - - - -	- - - - -
Intelligence _____		
Maturational level _____		
Organic signs _____		

Note.   Check off all categories that apply. TAT = Thematic Apperception Test; m = male; f = female. From *Thematic Apperception Test Short Form,* by L. Bellak, 1955, Larchmont, NJ: CPS. Copyright 1955 by Leopold Bellak, MD. Adapted with permission.

Six Decades of the Thematic Apperception Test

In the first 2 decades following the publication of Murray's (1943) TAT, several authors published full-length books presenting their own method of scoring the TAT that clinical psychologists can use in their psychological test battery diagnostic assessments (Arnold, 1951, 1962; Aron, 1949; Bellak, 1954; Henry, 1947; Shneidman, 1952; Stein, 1955, 1981; Tomkins, 1947). Research investigation of the TAT had great success in the objective scoring of different needs in Murray's system, such as the work of McClelland (1955; McClelland, Atkinson, Clark, & Lowell, 1953) on the achievement motive and of Atkinson, Hyns, and Veroff (1954) on the need for affiliation (also see Winter, chap. 9, this volume).

Shneidman, Joel, and Little (1951) attracted a lively attention to the TAT with the publication of the TAT protocol of a young man that Shneidman sent to a number of different authors who had developed their own TAT scoring system. The TAT protocol was sent to these authors without giving them any identifying information on the author of the protocol and these TAT analyses were published in *Thematic Test Analysis,* followed by a history and background of this actual protocol (also see Shneidman, chap. 7, this volume).

Bellak's contribution to Shneidman's book and the success of Bellak's (1954) own book illustrating his multidimensional TAT approach influenced a large number of researchers who investigated different dimensions of his scoring system in the late 1950s, 1960s, and 1970s. These were studies of the following dimensions: main hero (Friedman, 1957), significant conflicts (Abrams, 1977; Epstein, 1962), nature of anxieties (Mandler,

Lindzey, & Crouch, 1957), main defenses (Blum, 1964; Cramer & Carter, 1978; Dias, 1976; Haworth, 1963; Heath, 1958; Heilbrun, 1977), moral judgment and superego (Kohlberg, 1969; Shore, Massimo, & Mack, 1964), and integration of the ego and general ego functions (Bachrach & Peterson, 1976; Born, 1975; Dies, 1968; Dudek, 1975; Johnson & Kilmann, 1975; Morval, 1977; Pine, 1960; Stolorow, 1973; Weissman, 1964; Wyatt, 1958).

In the decades of the 1980s and 1990s, contemporary psychodynamic theory developed in three primary areas with parallel developments in TAT research: (a) the analysis of internal conflict expressed in drive–defense constellations developed within mainstream psychoanalysis, (b) the British object relations school developed Sigmund Freud's ego function of interpersonal object relations into a primary approach to treatment, and (c) Kohut (1971, 1977) developed S. Freud's early work on narcissism and the ego function of the capacity for self- and object representation.

Consequently, Bellak's comprehensive scoring system further emphasizes these three important developments. Most notably, within mainstream ego psychology on defense and ego analysis, there is Cramer's (1991b, 1996) empirical scoring system for defense mechanisms on the TAT. Cramer only focused on the three defenses of denial, projection, and identification. Her work shows that these three main defenses characterize the three main stages of child development from preschool years (denial), elementary school years (projection), and high school years (identification). This developmental shift in defenses can also successfully differentiate more severe psychiatric disorders that rely more on denial and projection from more neurotic and adaptive levels of functioning that rely more on identification (Cramer, 1996).

The development of the British object relations school of psychoanalysis is best represented in TAT research in the object relations scoring systems of McAdams (1980), Thomas and Dudek (1985), and the extensive work of Drew Westen and his colleagues (Berends, Westen, Leigh, & Silbert, 1990; Leigh, 1992; Westen, 1991; Westen, Lohr, Silk, Gold, & Kerber, 1990; Westen, Ludolph, Lerner, Ruffins, & Wiss, 1990). It is also well illustrated in two research and clinical volumes of Francis Kelly (1996, 1997). The Kohut direction of self-psychology or the study of normal and pathological narcissism has not resulted in any development in TAT scoring. However, pioneering adult TAT case presentations of narcissistic patients have been published by Francoise Brelet-Foulard (Brelet, 1981, 1983, 1986; Brelet-Foulard, 1994) in France and Shulman, McGarthy, and Ferguson (1988) in the United States. I (Abrams, 1993/1995) have published narcissistic child and adolescent Children's Apperception Test (CAT) and TAT case presentations.

Related to the area of interpersonal object relations is the field of family therapy, in which TAT family studies have been contributed by Ferreira and Winter (1965); Ferreira, Winter, and Poindexter (1966); Minuchin (1967); Werner, Stabenau, and Pollin (1970); and Winter and Ferreira (1969, 1970). Perhaps the most important application of the family systems perspective to TAT research is the communication deviance (CD) scoring approach first documented by Jones (1977), which has continued to be developed in a host of valuable research studies (Doane, Miklowitz, Oranchak, & Flores de Apodaca, 1989; Doane & Mintz, 1987; Goldstein, 1988; Karon & Widener, 1994; Miklowitz et al., 1986; Miklowitz, Velligan, Goldstein, & Neuchterlein, 1991; Rund, 1989; Sharav, 1991; Velligan, Goldstein, Nuechterlein, Miklowitz, & Ranlett, 1990).

Given the fact that the three pivotal approaches to psychotherapy are psychoanalytic therapy, family therapy, and behavior therapy, psychologists have long awaited a contribution to TAT research and clinical diagnosis from the field of behavior therapy. Finally, there has appeared the well-conducted research articles on the personal problem-solving TAT scoring approach by George Ronan and his colleagues (Ronan, Colavito, & Hammontree, 1993; Ronan, Date, & Weisbrod, 1995), which is an important new development in the field.

Other developments in the last 2 decades of TAT research have been the extension of the TAT into diagnostic studies of borderline disorders (Rogoff, 1985; Rosoff, 1988; Westen, Klepser, et al., 1991; Westen, Lohr, et al., 1990; Westen, Ludolph, Block, Wixom, & Wiss, 1991; Westen, Ludolph, et al., 1990), the aforementioned work on narcissistic disorders (Abrams, 1993/1995; Brelet, 1981, 1983, 1986; Brelet-Foulard, 1994, 1995; Harder, 1979; Shulman et al., 1988), attention deficit disorder (Bellak & Abrams, 1997; Costantino, Colon-Malgady, Malgady, & Perez, 1991), mental retardation (Hurley & Sovner, 1985), substance abuse (Brelet, 1988; Cabal Bravo et al., 1990; Fassino et al., 1992; Wilson, Passik, Faude, Abrams, & Gordon, 1989), eating disorders (Williams, 1986), and trauma (Henderson, 1990; Hoffman & Kuperman, 1990; Stovall & Craig, 1990).

As psychologists look over the last 6 decades of the TAT, a pattern emerges: Each researcher chose to develop an objective scoring approach for a single dimension of personality organization, which tended to be a category that was already one of the 10 dimensions of Bellak's scoring system.

Value of a Contemporary Multidimensional Scoring System

The Bellak scoring system has always been presented as a "guide for clinical use" based on the major dimensions of personality organization from the common frameworks of contemporary theories of personality, psychopathology, and contemporary clinical practice. It is largely an integration of Murray's (1938) personology theory of need–press relationships and contemporary psychoanalytic or psychodynamic theory. It is also an open system that allows the clinician to include dimensions from other theories or to focus more clinical attention on 1 or 2 of the 10 categories, as in the examples of Cramer's (1991a, 1996) assessment of defense mechanisms or the Westen interpersonal object relations assessment (Kelly, 1996, 1997;

Westen, Klepser, et al., 1991; Westen, Lohr, et al., 1990; Westen, Ludolph, et al., 1990, 1991).

Clinicians have found that although the Bellak system takes some time to learn and requires familiarity with contemporary understanding of personality development and psychiatric disorders, the Bellak short form can be checked off in a little over 30 minutes for the standard sequence of 10 TAT stories. The 10 categories help to remind the clinician of the important areas or "axes" of personality organization and psychopathology that lead to the best level of personality assessment and clinical diagnosis in concert with the mental status evaluation. Another reason that the Bellak scoring system has remained the predominant method of TAT assessment is due to the fact that the *Diagnostic and Statistical Manual of Mental Disorders* (4th ed.; American Psychiatric Association, 1994) also calls for a multiaxial clinical assessment approach.

This multidimensional "systems" view of personality organization is open and inclusive rather than closed and exclusive. S. Freud similarly believed in an open system of personality assessment, to which he continued to add new dimensions with the advances of his psychoanalytic theory and clinical experience. In the days when schizophrenia tended to be viewed unidimensionally, Bellak (1948, 1958, 1969) pioneered a general systems diagnostic approach to consider subtypes from similar multidimensional perspectives. In this way, the Bellak scoring system resembles the multitrait assessment of human functioning advocated for personality assessment with the TAT by McAdams (1995).

As new research studies are conducted, new scoring variables are discovered, new understandings of clinical disorders are communicated (e.g., work on attention deficit, borderline, and narcissistic disorders), and psychologists are asked to do evaluations of individuals of other cultures or in forensic settings, the method of TAT scoring may need to be updated, revised, and further developed to encompass these advances. It is for this reason that the Bellak text continues to be updated and revised every few years. The main criticism of the Bellak scoring system is that it is a clinical checklist approach to the TAT, a way of summarizing themes and noting different areas of functioning, as in a good clinical mental status evaluation rather than an empirically based research scoring system.

In the 1997 edition of *The T.A.T., C.A.T., and S.A.T. in Clinical Use,* Bellak and Abrams delineated where the many research studies using objective scoring variables contributed to a more empirical scoring of many of the 10 categories of Bellak's TAT scoring system. Most notably there is Cramer's (1991a, 1991b, 1996) scoring of defenses and the Westen (1991) scoring of Bellak's interpersonal object relations category. Although any one of Bellak's 10 scoring dimensions may provide a fairly good clinical assessment of TAT responses (Abrams, 1993), psychologists should question whether even a 4-part purely object relations approach, such as that of Westen, is too one sided for clinical use.

In a survey study, Rossini and Moretti (1997) sent a questionnaire to 130 clinical psychology doctoral programs and asked the professors responsible for teaching the initial graduate-level assessment course directly involving the TAT to check which on a long list of books, chapters, and journal articles on the TAT they either require or recommend for the students in their course. Of the 39% who returned the questionnaire, over a third required or recommended the Bellak text at the top of the list, followed by Murray's (1943) TAT manual in close second.

Rossini and Moretti's (1997) article provides a list of publications the professors surveyed found most useful for their students. Rossini and Moretti also cited publications that they believed should be placed on required or recommended lists that were not mentioned by the professors and which should be ranked higher in their opinion. For example, they stated that their own teacher used Henry's (1956) interpretive TAT book instead of Bellak's book in their graduate training, which they preferred for the "psychodynamically based outline of each card's utility in terms of manifest content and inferred latent psychodynamic stimulus value" (p. 396). However, Henry's book was required by only 11% and recommended by 18% of the respondents. They recommended Holt's (1978b) chapter, "A Normative Guide to the Use of the TAT Cards" and Schafer's (1958) journal article titled "How Was This Story Told," even though only 5% of the respondents had these on their required list. Finally, they recommended a chapter by Karon (1981) and journal articles by Hartman (1970) and Peterson (1990), which were not even on the list of required or recommended readings. Henry's (1956) valuable TAT book, in my view, is very heavily based on the impressionistic psychoanalytic symbolism of different cards of that period in time. This makes the book rather dated. Henry's interpretive method is now difficult to learn and apply to TAT protocols for the language of current clinical test reports.

As Rossini and Moretti (1997) recommended, if Henry's book is used as the only text in TAT teaching of clinical psychology doctoral students, it must be revised to incorporate further advances in personality assessment and the large research tradition since 1956 of more than a thousand empirical studies using objective scoring methods. Rossini and Moretti (1997) further recommended that "unless a quantified scoring system is used and appropriate normative data are publicly available" (p. 395), the TAT "should never be called the Thematic Apperception 'Test' " (p. 395). This is a reasonable proviso, and one Murray and Bellak themselves had considered earlier, Murray originally referring to the TAT as a "projective interview technique" and Bellak entitling his test to be used with older people, the Senior Apperception Technique (also see Gieser & Stein, chap. 17, this volume).

Nevertheless, there is the rather extensive early normative TAT literature using objective scoring (Eron, 1950; Murstein, 1972; Neman, Brown, & Sells, 1973; Neman, Neman, & Sells, 1974; Sells, Cox, & Chatman, 1967; Zubin, Eron, & Schumer, 1965) and the later extensive work of Zhang, Xu, Cai, and Chen (1993) in China; Shentoub et al. (1990) in France; and Avila Espada (1983, 1986, 1990) in Spain. In three full-length books, Avila Espada, for example, reported large-scale normative TAT studies in which he used a large list of objective scoring variables. Examples of these variables are number of words in a story, mention of overt aggression, frequency of different themes, presence of story-ending statements, and presence of bizarre or peculiar verbalizations. Avila Espada's work demonstrates the capacity for the TAT to meet the criteria of objective test construction (standardized administration; standard card sequence; objective scoring; established age, socioeconomic, cultural, and other norms; adequate test reliability; and validity). Further normative research will bring psychologists closer to the high standard of Exner's empirically based Rorschach scoring system.

Replacing Murray's Manual

Finally, Rossini and Moretti (1997) recommended the publication of a workbook to replace Murray's (1943) TAT manual, which is sold along with the TAT cards. They called for a workbook that uses an objective scoring system based on contemporary personality theory, reports established age and other norms, and includes a series of graduated full-length TAT protocols. In addition, they declared that it should be officially "endorsed by the Society for Personality Assessment or some other national group" (Rossini & Moretti, 1997, p. 395).

Indeed, every author who developed their own scoring scheme for the Rorschach, TAT, or projective drawings—from Exner (1994) for the Rorshach plates, Hammer (1985) for the House-Tree-Person Drawing Test, or Stein (1955/1981) or Bellak for the TAT—would love to have their work officially accepted as the standard manual or text for a particular test by a professional specialist society or by the entire American Psychological Association. I suggest that the use of a standard administration, standard card sequence, and standard scoring approach with increasing objective scoring research studies; establishment of age, gender, socioeconomic, culture, and other norms; and reliability and validity studies will help to bring the TAT closer to this goal. However, I believe that the TAT is richer for the ever-increasing availability of a variety of scoring schemes, just as the more empirically based Exner–Rorschach approach continues to co-exist with valuable content-based scoring systems (Aronow & Reznikoff, 1976) or more psychoanalytic based systems (Schafer, 1954).

Although some psychologists are understandably partisan to the Bellak TAT scoring system, it will hopefully remain as only one of several approaches to clinical assessment with thematic tests. As Bellak and Abrams (1997) emphasized in their TAT textbook, every psychologist should be familiar with the many valuable scoring systems for thematic tests from the four major schools of psychotherapy—psychoanalytic conflict-focused psychotherapy (Bellak, 1954; Cramer, 1991a; Henry, 1956; Holt, 1978a, 1978b; Pine, 1960; Schafer, 1958; Stein, 1981), interpersonal object relations psychotherapy (Kelly, 1996, 1997; Westen, Klepser, et al., 1991; Westen, Lohr, et al., 1990; Westen, Ludolph, et al., 1990, 1991), family therapy (Jones, 1977; Karon & Widener, 1994; Singer & Wynne, 1966), and behavioral–cognitive therapy (Ronan et al., 1993, 1995). As previously noted, although family therapy is actually related to the object relations approach to psychotherapy, there needs to be a better understanding of family systems theory in scoring the interpersonal object relations of TAT dimensions.

The interesting contributions of Carl Jung to dream interpretation, word association, stages of the individuation process, and other areas have never, to my knowledge, been applied to TAT scoring. Murray and Christiana Morgan were both influenced by Jung and tried to develop a Jungian TAT II based on archetypes (see N. Murray, preface, this volume). The recognition of complexes of personality needs and motivations in Murray's scoring scheme for the TAT indirectly reflects Jung's influence. Hopefully, someone will develop a way to score the TAT specifically using concepts from Jung's analytic psychology.

The future of TAT assessment will remain on a good course with continued research on ways to objectify the various personality dimensions for which it provides data. Metaphorically speaking, the TAT is a big tent under which there is plenty of room for psychologists of all theoretical persuasions.

References

Abrams, D. M. (1977). *Conflict resolution in children's fantasy storytelling: A test of Erikson's theory and of the culture-enculturation hypothesis*. Unpublished doctoral dissertation, Columbia University.

Abrams, D. M. (1993). Pathological narcissism in an eight-year-old boy: An example of Bellak's TAT and CAT diagnostic system. *Psychoanalytic Psychology, 10*, 573–591. (French translation published 1995, *Psychologie Clinique et Projective, 1*, 245–267)

American Psychiatric Association. (1994). *Diagnostic and statistical manual of mental disorders* (4th ed.). Washington, DC: Author.

Arnold, M. (1951). Analysis of John Doe. In E. S. Shneidman (Ed.), *Thematic test analysis* (pp. 63–72). New York: Grune & Stratton.

Arnold, M. B. (1962). *Story sequence analysis*. New York: Columbia University Press.

Aron, B. (1949). *A manual for analysis of the Thematic Apperception Test*. Berkeley, CA: Willis E. Berg.

Aronow, E., & Reznikoff, M. (1976). *Rorschach content interpretation*. New York: Grune & Stratton.

Atkinson, J. W., Hyns, R. W., & Veroff, J. (1954). The effect of experimental arousal of the affiliative motive in thematic apperception. *Journal of Abnormal and Social Psychology, 49*, 405–410.

Avila Espada, A. (1983). *El Test de Apercepcion Tematica de H. A. Murray en la poblacion Espanola: Estudio normativo y analisis para una adaptacion* [The Thematic Apperception Test of H. A. Murray in the Spanish population] (Vols. 1–2). Madrid, Spain: Editorial de la Universidad Complutense.

Avila Espada, A. (1986). *Manual operativo del T.A.T* [Operational TAT manual]. Madrid, Spain: Editorial Piramide.

Avila Espada, A. (1990). *Fundamentos empiricos del Test de Apercepcion Tematica* [Empirical foundations of the Thematic Apperception Test]. Madrid, Spain: Editorial Piramide.

Bachrach, R., & Peterson, R. A. (1976). Test–retest reliability among three locus of control measures for children. *Perceptual and Motor Skills, 43*, 260–262.

Bellak, L. (1944). The concept of projection: An experimental investigation and study of the concept. *Psychiatry, 7*, 353–370.

Bellak, L. (1948). *Dementia praecox*. New York: Grune & Stratton.

Bellak, L. (1950a). A further experimental investigation of projection by means of hypnosis. In L. W. Crafts, T. C. Schneirla, E. E. Robinson, & R. W. Gilbert (Eds.), *Recent experiments in psychology* (pp. 33–39). New York: McGraw-Hill.

Bellak, L. (1950b). Thematic apperception: Failures and the defenses. *Transactions of the New York Academy of Science* [Series II], *12*, 112–126.

Bellak, L. (1950c). Projection and the Thematic Apperception Test. In L. W. Crafts, T. C. Schneirla, E. E. Robinson, & R. W. Gilbert (Eds.), *Recent experiments in psychology* (pp. 21–27). New York: McGraw-Hill.

Bellak, L. (1950d). Thematic apperception: Failures and the defenses. *Transactions of the New York Academy of Science* [Series II], *12, 112–126.*

Bellak, L. (1954). *The T.A.T. and C.A.T. in clinical use.* New York: Grune & Stratton.

Bellak, L. (1955). *Thematic Apperception Test short form.* Larchmont, NY: CPS.

Bellak, L. (1958). *Schizophrenia: A review of the syndrome.* New York: Grune & Stratton.

Bellak, L. (1969). *The schizophrenia syndrome.* New York: Grune & Stratton.

Bellak, L. & Abrams, D. M. (1997). *The T.A.T., C.A.T., and S.A.T. in clinical use.* Needham Heights, MA: Allyn & Bacon.

Berends, A., Westen, D., Leigh, J., & Silbert, D. (1990). Assessing affect-tone of relationship in paradigms from TAT and interview data. *Psychological Assessment, 2*, 329–332.

Blum, G. S. (1964). Defense preferences among university students in Denmark, France, Germany and Israel. *Journal of Projective Techniques and Personality Assessment, 28*, 13–19.

Born, M. (1975). Pour une approche quantitative de fonctions de l'ego dans le TAT [Attempts at a quantitative approach to ego functions in the TAT]. *Revue de Psychologie et des Sciences de l'Education, 10*, 435–444.

Brelet, F. (1981). A propos du narcissisme dans le T.A.T. [On narcissism in the TAT]. *Psychologie Francaise, 26*, 24–37.

Brelet, F. (1983). Le T.A.T. et narcissisme: Perspectives dynamiques et economiques [TAT and narcissism: Dynamic and economic perspectives]. *Psychologie Francaise, 28*, 119–123.

Brelet, F. (1986). *Le T.A.T.: Fantasme et situation projective: Narcissisme, fonctionnement limite, depression* [The TAT: Fantasy and the projective situation: Narcissism, borderline functioning, depression]. Paris, France: Dunod.

Brelet, F. (1988). *Le T.A.T.: Fantasme et situation projective: Une application clinique: Le T.A.T. chez l'alcoholique* [The TAT: Fantasy and the projective situation: A clinical application of the TAT with the alcoholic]. Unpublished doctoral dissertation, University of Paris X, Nanterre, France.

Brelet-Foulard, F. (1994). Expression of narcissistic fantasy in the TAT. *Rorschachiana, 19*, 97–112.

Brelet-Foulard, F. (1995). En echo: Réponse à l'article de David M. Abrams [In echo: Response to the article by David M. Abrams]. *Psychologie Clinique et Projective, 1*, 269–274.

Cabal Bravo, J. C., Bobes Garcia, J., Vazquez Fernandez, A., Gonzalez-Quiros Corujo, P., Bousono Garcia, M., Garcia Prieto, A., & Garcia-Portilla, P. (1990). TAT: Psicodiagnostico en pacientes heroinomanos [Thematic Apperception Test: Psychodiagnosis in heroin-dependent patients]. *Actas Luso-Españolas de Neurologia, Psiquiatria y Ciencias Afines, 18*, 1–6.

Costantino, G., Colon-Malgady, G., Malgady, R. G., & Perez, A. (1991). Assessment of attention deficit disorder using a thematic apperceptive technique. *Journal of Personality Assessment, 57*, 87–95.

Cramer, P. (1991a). Anger and the use of defense mechanisms in college students. *Journal of Personality, 59*, 39–55.

Cramer, P. (1991b). *The development of defense mechanisms: Theory, research, and assessment.* New York: Springer-Verlag.

Cramer, P. (1996). *Storytelling, narrative, and the Thematic Apperception Test.* New York: Guilford Press.

Cramer, P., & Carter, T. (1978). The relationship between sexual identification and the use of defense mechanisms. *Journal of Personality Assessment, 42*, 63–73.

Dias, B. (1976). *Les mecanismes de defense dans la genese des normes de conduite: Etude experimentale basee sur le Thematic Apperception Test (T.A.T.)* [Defense mechanisms in the etiology of behavioral norms: Experimental study based on the Thematic Apperception Test (TAT)]. Fribourg, Switzerland: Editions Universitaires.

Dies, R. R. (1968). Development of a projective measure of perceived locus of control. *Journal of Projective Techniques and Personality Assessment, 32*, 487–490.

Doane, J. A., Miklowitz, D. J., Oranchak, E., & Flores de Apodaca, R. (1989). Parental communication deviance and schizophrenia: A cross-cultural comparison of Mexican- and Anglo-Americans. *Journal of Abnormal Psychology, 98*, 487–490.

Doane, J. A., & Mintz, J. (1987). Communication deviance in adolescence and adulthood: A longitudinal study. *Psychiatry, 50*, 5–13.

Dudek, S. Z. (1975). Regression in the service of the ego in young children. *Journal of Personality Assessment, 39*, 369–376.

Epstein, S. (1962). The measurement of drive and conflict in humans: Theory and experiment. In M. Jones (Ed.), *Nebraska Symposium on Motivation* (pp. 11–25). Lincoln: University of Nebraska Press.

Eron, L. D. (1950). A normative study of the Thematic Apperception Test. *Psychological Monographs, 64*(9, Whole No. 315).

Exner, J. E. (1994). *The Rorschach: A comprehensive system* (Vol. 1). New York: Wiley.

Fassino, S., Scarso, G., Barbero, L., Taylor, J., Pezzini, F., & Furian, P. M. (1992). The image of self and of the environment in drug abusers: A comparative study using the TAT. *Drug and Alcohol Dependence, 30*, 253–261.

Ferreira, A. J., & Winter, W. D. (1965). Family interaction and decision-making. *Archives of General Psychiatry, 13*, 214–223.

Ferreira, A. J., Winter, W. D., & Poindexter, E. (1966). Some interactional variables in normal and abnormal families. *Family Process, 5*, 60–75.

Freud, A. (1965). *Normality and pathology of childhood.* New York: International Universities Press.

Freud, S. (1923). The ego and the id. In J. Strachey (Ed. & Trans.), *The standard edition of the complete psychological works of Sigmund Freud* (Vol. 19, pp. 12–66). London: Hogarth Press.

Friedman, I. (1957). Characteristics of the Thematic Apperception Test heroes of normal, psychoneurotic, and paranoid schizophrenic subjects. *Journal of Projective Techniques, 21*, 372–376.

Goldstein, M. J. (1988). Family factors that antedate the onset of schizophrenia and related disorders: The results of a fifteen year prospective longitudinal study. *Acta Psychiatrica Scandinavia, 71*, 7–18.

Hammer, E. F. (1985). The House-Tree-Person Drawing Test. In C. S. Newmark (Ed.), *Major psychological assessment instruments* (pp. 135–164). Boston: Allyn & Bacon.

Harder, D. W. (1979). The assessment of ambitious–narcissistic character style with three projective tests: The early memories, TAT, and Rorschach. *Journal of Personality Assessment, 43*, 23–32.

Hartman, A. H. (1970). A basic TAT set. *Journal of Projective Techniques, 34*, 391–396.

Haworth, M. R. (1963). A schedule for the analysis of C.A.T. responses. *Journal of Projective Techniques and Personality Assessment, 27*, 181–184.

Heath, D. H. (1958). Projective tests as measures of defensive activity. *Journal of Projective Techniques, 22*, 284–292.

Heilbrun, A. B. (1977). The influence of defensive styles upon the predictive validity of the Thematic Apperception Test. *Journal of Personality Assessment, 41*, 486–491.

Henderson, O. (1990). The object relations of sexually abused girls. *Melanie Klein and Object Relations, 8*, 63–76.

Henry, W. E. (1947). Thematic Apperception Test in the study of culture personality relations. *Genetic Psychology Monographs, 35*.

Henry, W. E. (1956). *The analysis of fantasy: The thematic apperception technique in the study of personality.* New York: Wiley. (Reprinted in 1973 by Krieger, Huntington, NY)

Hoffman, S., & Kuperman, N. (1990). Indirect treatment of traumatic psychological experiences: The use of TAT cards. *American Journal of Psychotherapy, 44*, 107–115.

Holt, R. R. (1978a). *Methods in clinical psychology: Projective assessments* (Vol. 1). New York: Plenum Press.

Holt, R. R. (1978b). A normative guide to the use of the TAT cards. In R. R. Holt (Ed.), *Methods in clinical psychology: Projective assessments* (Vol. 1, pp. 77–123). New York: Plenum Press.

Hurley, A. D., & Sovner, R. (1985). The use of the Thematic Apperception Test in mentally retarded persons. *Psychiatric Aspects of Mental Retardation Reviews, 4*, 9–12.

Johnson, B. L., & Kilmann, P. B. (1975). Prediction of locus of control orientation from the Thematic Apperception Test. *Journal of Clinical Psychology, 31*, 547–548.

Jones, J. E. (1977). Patterns of transactional style deviance in the TATs of parents of schizophrenics. *Family Process, 16*, 327–337.

Karon, B. P. (1981). The Thematic Apperception Test (TAT). In A. I. Rabin (Ed.), *Assessment with projective techniques* (pp. 85–120). New York: Springer.

Karon, B. P., & Widener, A. J. (1994). Is there really a schizophrenic parent? *Psychoanalytic Psychology, 11*, 47–61.

Kelly, F. D. (1996). *The assessment of object relations phenomena in younger children: Rorschach and TAT measures.* Springfield, IL: Charles C Thomas.

Kelly, F. D. (1997). *The assessment of object relations phenomena in adolescents: TAT and Rorschach measures.* Mahwah, NJ: Erlbaum.

Kohlberg, L. (1969). *Stages in the development of moral thought and action.* New York: Holt.

Kohut, H. (1971). *The analysis of the self.* New York: International Universities Press.

Kohut, H. (1977). *The restoration of the self.* New York: International Universities Press.

Leigh, J. (1992). The assessment of complexity of representations of people using TAT and interview data. *Journal of Personality, 60*, 809–837.

Mandler, G., Lindzey, G., & Crouch, R. G. (1957). Thematic Apperception Test: Indices of anxiety in relation to test anxiety. *Educational Psychological Measurements, 17*, 466–474.

McAdams, D. P. (1980). A thematic coding system for the intimacy motive. *Journal of Research in Personality, 14*, 413–432.

McAdams, D. P. (1995). What do we know when we know a person? *Journal of Personality, 63*, 364–396.

McClelland, D. C. (1955). *Studies in motivation.* New York: Appleton-Century-Crofts.

McClelland, D. C., Atkinson, J. E., Clark, R. A., & Lowell, E. L. (1953). *The achievement motive.* New York: Irvington.

Miklowitz, D. J., Strachan, A. M., Goldstein, M. J., Doane, J. A., Snyder, K. S., Hogarty, G. E., & Falloon, I. R. (1986). Expression emotion and communication deviance in the families of schizophrenics. *Journal of Abnormal Psychology, 95*, 60–66.

Miklowitz, D. J., Velligan, D. I., Goldstein, M. J., & Neuchterlein, K. H. (1991). Communication deviance in families of schizophrenic and manic patients. *Journal of Abnormal Psychology, 100*, 163–173.

Minuchin, S. (1967). *Families of the slums—An exploration of their structure and treatment.* New York: Basic Books.

Morval, M. (1977). *Le TAT et les fonctions de moi* [The TAT and ego functions]. Montreal, Quebec, Canada: Presses de l'Universite de Montreal.

Murray, H. A. (Ed.). (1938). *Explorations in personality: A clinical and experimental study of fifty men of college age.* New York: Oxford University Press.

Murray, H. A. (1943). *Thematic Apperception Test: Manual.* Cambridge, MA: Harvard University Press.

Murray, H. A., & Bellak, L. (1941). *Interpretation categories for the Thematic Apperception Test.* Unpublished manuscript, Harvard Psychological Clinic, Cambridge, MA.

Murray, H. A., & Bellak, L. (1955). *Thematic Apperception Test blank.* Unpublished mimeograph, Harvard Psychological Clinic, Cambridge, MA.

Murstein, B. I. (1972). Normative written TAT responses for a college sample. *Journal of Personality Assessment, 36*, 109–147.

Neman, R. S., Brown, T. S., & Sells, S. B. (1973). Language and adjustment scales for the Thematic Apperception Test for children 6–11 years: A report on the development and standardization of objective scoring procedures for five cards of the TAT used in the

Health Examination Survey of children 6–11 years of age. *Vital and Health Statistics* (Series 2), No. 3, 58–73.

Neman, R. S., Neman, J. F., & Sells, S. B. (1974). Language and adjustment scales for the Thematic Apperception Test for youths 12–17 years. *Vital and Health Statistics* (Series 2), No. 62, 1–84.

Peterson, C. A. (1990). Administration of the Thematic Apperception Test: Contributions of psychoanalytic psychotherapy. *Journal of Contemporary Psychotherapy, 20*, 191–200.

Pine, F. (1960). A manual for rating drive content in the Thematic Apperception Test. *Journal of Projective Techniques, 24*, 32–45.

Rogoff, T. L. (1985). TAT disturbances of thinking in borderline personality disorder: Differential diagnosis of inpatient borderlines from schizophrenics, schizotypals, and other personality disorders. *Dissertation Abstracts International, 46*, 658–659.

Ronan, G. F., Colavito, V. A., & Hammontree, S. R. (1993). Personal problem-solving system for scoring TAT responses: Preliminary validity and reliability data. *Journal of Personality Assessment, 61*, 28–40.

Ronan, G. F., Date, A. L., & Weisbrod, M. (1995). Personal problem-solving scoring of the TAT: Sensitivity to training. *Journal of Personality Assessment, 64*, 119–131.

Rosoff, A. L. (1988). Thematic Apperception Test characteristics and the psychotherapy of schizophrenic patients: A study of pretreatment patient *variables* and psychotherapy process. *Dissertation Abstracts International, 48*, 2108.

Rossini, E. D., & Moretti, R. J. (1997). Thematic Apperception Test (TAT) interpretation: Practice recommendations from a survey of clinical psychology doctoral programs accredited by the American Psychological Association. *Professional Psychology: Research and Practice, 28*, 393–398.

Rund, B. R. (1989). Communication deviances in parents of schizophrenics. *Family Process, 25*, 133–147.

Schafer, R. (1954). *Psychoanalytic interpretation in Rorschach testing*. New York: Grune & Stratton.

Schafer, R. (1958). How was this story told? *Journal of Projective Techniques, 22*, 181–210.

Sells, S. B., Cox, S. H., & Chatman, L. R. (1967). Scales of language development for the TAT. *Vital and Health Statistics* (Series 2), No. 2, 171–172.

Sharav, D. (1991). Assessing adoptive parents using a combined individual and interaction procedure. In E. D. Hibbs (Ed.), *Adoption: International perspectives* (pp. 73–89). Madison, CT: International Universities Press.

Shentoub, V., Azoulay, C., Bailly-Salin, M.-J., Benfredj, K., Boekholt, M., Brelet, F., Chabert, C., Chretien, M., Emmanuelli, M., Martin, M., Monin, E., Peruchon, M., & Serviere, A. (1990). *Manuel d'utilisation du T.A.T. (approche psychanalytique)* [Manual for the use of the TAT (psychoanalytic approach)]. Paris, France: Dunod.

Shneidman, E. S. (1952). *The Make-a-Picture-Story Test (MAPS)*. New York: The Psychological Corporation.

Shneidman, E. S., Joel, W., & Little, K. B. (1951). *Thematic test analysis*. New York: Grune & Stratton.

Shore, M. F., Massimo, J. L., & Mack, R. (1964). The relationship between levels of guilt and unsocialized behavior. *Journal of Projective and Personality Assessment, 28*, 346–349.

Shulman, D. G., McGarthy, E. C., & Ferguson, G. R. (1988). The projective assessment of narcissism: Development, reliability and validity of the N-P. *Psychoanalytic Psychology, 5*, 285–297.

Singer, M., & Wynne, L. (1966). Principles for scoring communication deviances in parents of schizophrenics: Rorschach and TAT scoring manuals. *Psychiatry, 29*, 260–288.

Stein, M. I. (1981). *The Thematic Apperception Test: An introductory manual for its clinical use with adult males*. Cambridge, MA: Addison-Wesley. (Original work published 1955)

Stolorow, R. D. (1973). TAT coding system for the theme of voluntary control. *Catalog of Selected Documents in Psychology, 3*(51), 23–31.

Stovall, G., & Craig, R. J. (1990). Mental representations of physically and sexually abused latency-aged females. *Child Abuse & Neglect, 14*, 233–242.

Thomas, A. D., & Dudek, S. Z. (1985). Interpersonal affect in Thematic Apperception Test responses: A scoring system. *Journal of Personality Assessment, 49*, 30–36.

Tomkins, S. S. (1947). *The Thematic Apperception Test: The theory and technique of interpretation*. New York: Grune & Stratton.

Velligan, D. I., Goldstein, M. J., Nuechterlein, K. H., Miklowitz, D. J., & Ranlett, G. (1990). Can communication deviance be measured in a family problem-solving interaction? *Family Process, 29*, 213–226.

Weissman, S. (1964). Some indicators of acting out behavior from the Thematic Apperception Test. *Journal of Projective Techniques, 28*, 366–375.

Werner, M., Stabenau, J. R., & Pollin, W. (1970). Thematic Apperception Test method for the differentiation of families of schizophrenics, delinquents, and normals. *Journal of Abnormal and Social Psychology, 75*, 139–145.

Westen, D. (1991). Clinical assessment of object relations using the TAT. *Journal of Personality Assessment, 56*, 127–133.

Westen, D., Klepser, J., Ruffins, S. A., Silverman, M., Lifton, M., & Boekamp, J. (1991). Object relations in children and adolescents: The development of working representations. *Journal of Consulting and Clinical Psychology, 59*, 400–409.

Westen, D., Lohr, N., Silk, K. R., Gold, L., & Kerber, K. (1990). Object relations and social cognition in borderlines, major depressives, and normals: A Thematic Apperception Test analysis. *Psychological Assessment, 2*, 355–364.

Westen, D., Ludolph, P., Block, M. J., Wixom, J., & Wiss, F. C. (1991). Developmental history and object relations in psychiatrically disturbed adolescent girls. *American Journal of Psychiatry, 148*, 1419–1420.

Westen, D., Ludolph, P., Lerner, H., Ruffins, S., & Wiss, C. (1990). Object relations in borderline adolescents. *Journal of the American Academy of Child and Adolescent Psychiatry, 29*, 338–348.

Williams, E. L. (1986). Early recollection and Thematic Apperception Test responses of restricted anorexic, bulimic anorexic, and bulimic women. *Dissertation Abstracts International, 47*, 810.

Wilson, A., Passik, S. D., Faude, J., Abrams, J., & Gordon, E. (1989). A hierarchical model of opiate addiction: Failures of self-regulation as a central aspect of substance abuse. *Journal of Nervous and Mental Disease, 177*, 390–399.

Winter, W. D., & Ferreira, A. J. (1969). *Research in family interaction: Readings and commentary*. Palo Alto, CA: Science & Behavior Books.

Winter, W. D., & Ferreira, A. J. (1970). A factor analysis of family interaction measures. *Journal of Projective Techniques and Personality Assessment, 34*, 55–63.

Wyatt, F. (1958). A principle for the interpretation of fantasy. *Journal of Projective Techniques, 22*, 173–180.

Zhang, T., Xu, S., Cai, Z., & Chen, Z. (1993). Research on the Thematic Apperception Test: Chinese revision and its norm. *Acta Psychologica Scandinavica, 25*, 314–323.

Zubin, J., Eron, L. D., & Schumer, F. (1965). *An experimental approach to projective techniques*. New York: Wiley.

Part V ───────────────────────

Contemporary Developments

13

How the Test Lives On: Extensions of the Thematic Apperception Test Approach

David C. McClelland

Harry Murray and Christiana Morgan designed the Thematic Apperception Test (TAT) as a diagnostic tool that would enable the clinician to discover the deepest unconscious strivings and complexes that shape an individual's life. It is a more systematic way of collecting the fantasies in the daytime than Sigmund Freud, Carl Jung, and their followers collected from night-time dreams. Yet it has evolved over the years into something of greater importance for psychology even more than that. For throughout the history of psychology in the 20th century, the TAT approach has emphasized the importance of what people spontaneously think about as opposed to the mainstream emphasis on how they perceive, think, and act in response to a stimulus, a question, or an experimental intervention.

Although the TAT's influence on mainstream assumptions in psychology has so far not been great, I hope to show that as its approach evolved in various ways, a case for a revolutionary new approach to psychology may slowly be building up, involving the psychology of mental content. To provide evidence for such a bold assertion, I briefly review how the TAT approach has evolved in the study of human motivation, identifying themes in the life story, discovering cross-cultural themes, and shaping the behavioral event interview and the study of competencies.

Study of Human Motivation

Murray's (1938) great book, *Explorations in Personality,* is characterized not only by imaginative vigor but also by his insistence on the importance of motives, as separate and distinct from Gordon Allport's (1937) traits. Clearly, he felt that motives, many of them unconscious, are the key to understanding the nature of people and human civilization, just as Freud demonstrated. I strongly agree. Perhaps, as a minister's son, I am all too aware that professed motives in church on Sunday to be kind and generous are so different from less conscious motives shown in everyday life. Or maybe Scots like Immanual Kant, David Hume, William McDougall, Murray, and me are naturally inclined to believe that what people want is the main determinant of what happens in their lives.

At any rate, it gave me a small "aha" feeling to discover in Robinson's (1992) biography of Murray, *Love's Story Told,* that Murray was the product of a Scottish father and an English Babcock mother because I am the product of a Scottish grandfather and an English Babcock grandmother. In fact, Murray and I turned out to have a common ancestor eight generations back through the Babcocks—who tended to run to New England doctors and divines named Ichabod and Hezekiah with appropriately creative although generally religious imaginations. I have seen oil paintings of what turned out to be mutual Babcock relations in Murray's dining room, but I had never gotten around to asking him who they were. How amused he would have been to discover our genetic relationship! Our mutual fascination with unconscious motivation may be attributed not only to our similar cultural backgrounds but also perhaps to an obscure microgenetic molecule (Saudino & Plomin, 1996) determining a love for fantasy and the TAT.

What I wanted to do was prove that Murray was right—that motives are key and often unconscious determinants of behavior, they are independent of traits, and they are uniquely measurable with the TAT. Given my behaviorist training at Yale University, what happened next was predictable. We (Murray and I) aroused motives experimentally, starting with one even a behaviorist would recognize—namely, hunger—and checked to see what its effects might be on behaviors such as self-reports of hunger, perception of objects, or thematic apperception stories (Atkinson & McClelland, 1948). We found that only the TAT yielded unique effects (content shifts in the stories) that increased in linear fashion with increasing hours of food deprivation in men who were not aware that their hunger drive was being studied. For example, self-reports of how hungry the men were did increase in curvilinear fashion with length of food deprivation, but their self-reports were also influenced by whether it was time to eat or not. Thus, one could not rely on self-rated hunger as reflecting purely and uniquely the hunger motive as defined by hours of food deprivation. Obviously, social hunger—the joint product of time of day and physiological need—might be important for certain types of research, but it was not a pure index of a physiologically defined hunger motive. Only the TAT could provide that.

Having removed social sources of distortion from the responses reflecting hunger by using the TAT, we next set about removing sources of distortion from the way the responses were observed. Murray believed—as most experts did at the time, especially those with a medical background— that the best possible measure of the strength of a motive in a given individual is the pooled opinion of a group of expert and experienced judges. But we felt this introduced the possibility of bias on the part of the judges. A group of people could obviously come to a pooled agreement on how hungry a person was on the basis of self-ratings of hunger, speed of perception of food objects, and TAT stories, but the judgment could still be wrong as checked against the hours the person had been without food. In fact, such judgments were apt to be wrong because most psychologist judges, knowing of earlier work by Sanford (1937), would think that the hungrier a person was the more apt he or she would be to write about delicious things to eat—which is not true, as we discovered, unless they have voluntarily chosen not to eat, as in Sanford's study. To rely on such social judgments of hunger, it seemed to us, would be like pooling the estimates of the temperature of a room from a group of people with varying backgrounds and levels of clothing. They might agree on a temperature, but it could also be far from what the thermometer actually recorded.

So we wanted a pure measure of the unique effects of an aroused motive; we developed coding systems for these effects that were so carefully defined that they yielded high interjudge agreement. In this way, the bias and even the wisdom of judges was removed by insisting that scores for a motive be only the frequency with which various effects of the aroused motive in the stories could be identified using strict rules for coding their presence or absence. We reasoned further that if such experimentally aroused effects occurred in an individual's TAT in the absence of arousal, then that person would show evidence of being strong in that motive because he or she was responding as if aroused, even under ordinary circumstances. Thus, we developed scoring systems for such individual differences in responsiveness to motive arousal for what has become the Big Three motives—*n* Achievement, *n* Affiliation, and *n* Power—and later in the same way for other motivational or thematic characteristics (Smith, 1992).

Afterwards, Murray once accosted me and said, "I suppose you think Jesus Christ had the highest *n* Achievement of all. After all, he wanted to change the entire world." I replied,

> Actually we've never scored for *n* Achievement the sayings attributed to Him in the Bible. So I don't know what His level of *n* Achievement is—since that is the only evidence we accept for determining motive strength. However, I strongly suspect He would score higher on *n* Power. For I recall off hand two of his sayings: "Consider the lilies of the field, they toil not; neither do they spin, yet Solomon in all his glory was not arrayed like one of these," which could scarcely be scored for *n* Achievement. And He also said, "Be of good cheer because I have overcome the world" which would be scored for *n* Power.

I could see Murray was not happy with these comments because he still believed that the ultimate determination of the strength of a motive should depend on the pooled informed opinions of experts, not on some experimentally derived scoring system.

However, we felt we had a purer measure of a motive, unaffected by observer bias, that might be influenced by such nonmotivational factors as the participant's own statement that he or she had a strong need to achieve (McClelland, Atkinson, Clark, & Lowell, 1953). We found then and have repeatedly found since that the strength of the "pure" measure of a motive derived from the TAT does not correlate with a participant's own statements as to the strength of the same motive. In simpler terms, the TAT motives are unconscious in the sense that over a group of participants, there is no correlation between what is called the implicit TAT-based motives and the explicit commitments to those same motives. Despite numerous meta-analyses showing that the two types of measures correlate at near zero levels (see McClelland, Koestner, & Weinberger, 1989; and Spangler, 1992), psychologists continue to act as if things that have the same name should measure the same characteristic—but in this case, they do not.

So a TAT-based motive is not a trait in Allport's (1937) sense of showing consistent behavior, such as reporting consistently that one is high in the motive in question or behaving in ways that look like what the motive is promoting. For example, many observers have made the mistaken assumption that n Achievement should be related to achieving behavior, such as doing well in school—the preeminent form of achievement for American psychologists. Yet generally speaking, n Achievement does not promote getting good grades (McClelland, 1987) or doing well on most laboratory tasks (McClelland, 1987, 1995), yet it does promote performing better on challenging tasks (Atkinson, 1958) and learning how to do better at unscrambling words (McClelland, 1995).

Insisting on the importance of the pure TAT-based motives has been only partly accepted by other psychologists for several reasons. One is semantic. The term *motivation* literally covers anything that impels or moves one to action. So time of day can motivate because it can impel one to eat. Or a statement such as "I want to eat" can motivate because it leads a person to eat. But strictly speaking, neither of these "motivators" are pure motives because they are shaped by other variables instead of motives. In short, motivation (the impulse to act) is only partly determined by motives, and it is difficult to persuade psychologists to keep this distinction in mind, but theoretically it is of major importance.

Another reason for the failure of the notion of pure TAT-based motives to catch on is that many psychologists still firmly believe that the evidence shows that any measure based on a mere projective test like the TAT is unreliable and invalid (e.g., see Entwistle, 1972). Yet by this time, reliability of implicit motive measures has been demonstrated (Winter & Stewart, 1977) as well as their validity. An impressive volume of theoretical and empirical findings demonstrates that n Achievement through its promotion of entrepreneurship is the engine of economic growth (McClelland, 1961; McClelland & Winter, 1971), n Power is the key to political and managerial leadership (Winter, 1973, 1996), and n Affiliation in its various guises plays a major role in health, both mental and physical (see McClelland, 1989).

Although such studies describe how these three important unconscious motives in their pure form influence important kinds of social behavior, more recent research has begun to illustrate how the motives influence and derive from basic physiological processes. It has been known for some time that arousal of TAT-based pure motives releases hormones specific to the motive in question, that is, epinephrine and norepinephrine from the arousal of n Power (McClelland, Davidson, Saron, & Floor, 1980; McClelland, Maddocks, & McAdams, 1985; Steele, reported in McClelland,

1987), dopamine from the arousal of n Affiliation (McClelland, Patel, Stier, & Brown, 1987), and arginine vasopressin from the arousal of n Achievement (McClelland, 1995). An increase of these hormones, either from internal or external sources, is known to enhance memory (McGaugh, 1990). So situations that release such hormones, which may be referred to as incentives, are rewarding in the sense that they reinforce learning or memory for the behavior by the person or animal. The question then becomes, How does an achievement incentive, characterized by a moderately challenging task (Atkinson, 1958), release arginine vasopressin, which provides the physiological basis for sending a message to the brain that serves as a reward or reinforcer?

High levels of TAT-type achievement motivation in adulthood are associated with strong achievement training in early life (see McClelland, 1961) but not just with any type of achievement training. McClelland and Pilon (1983) found that only scheduled infant feeding and particularly severe toilet training were associated with high n Achievement in adulthood over 25 years later. What is peculiar about these parent practices to account for their leading to a connection with release of vasopressin, which is associated with achievement arousal in adulthood (McClelland, 1995)? One possibility, currently speculative, derives from the known fact that injury to an organism, animal or human, releases vasopressin, which is an antidiuretic, the evolutionary function of which is to control loss of fluid in case of bleeding from a wound.

So one can imagine that inappropriately spanking a 12-month-old child for spilling urine could provide the unconditioned stimulus for the release of vasopressin, which has the desired effect of stopping urine flow. If the spanking is accompanied by repeated urgings to do better, to hold on to the urine, and to deposit it in the right place, then that could become the conditioned stimulus, which in time whenever it recurs would release vasopressin. Because such a punitively conditioned response is acquired early at a nearly preverbal stage, it would be hard to extinguish (McClelland, 1942) and could well last into adulthood.

Although much research remains to be conducted to verify whether such events actually occur, there is enough circumstantial evidence here to suggest an explanation for how basic human motives can become established unconsciously at an early period in life, just as Freud contended. Needless to say, I am not arguing that this is the only way or the only time in life when an achievement motive can be acquired because there is ample evidence of shifts in motive strengths that cannot be traced to childhood (McClelland & Winter, 1971; Veroff, Depner, Kulka, & Douvan, 1980). But at any rate, clearly TAT-based motives have been tied much more closely to biological processes than more complexly determined motives such as conscious desires for various goals.

Study of Themes in Life Stories

Fantasy for the psychoanalysts is a place for discovering themes that characterize aspects of the human condition—themes that are often reflected in popular myths. The discovery of the Oedipus complex is a classic example. Murray continued this tradition in using the TAT and identified the Icarus complex, the story of a young man who flew too high toward the sun on feathered wings stuck together with wax, which melted as he neared the sun, so that he fell into the sea. In examining the TAT fantasies of women threatened with death by cancer, Greenberger (see McClelland 1963a) found evidence for the existence of a complex named for Persephone, who was carried off underground by her demon lover, Hades, and finally escaped to bring joy to the earth in a life-enhancing way. That is, the women threatened with death wrote stories more often about being carried away by an illicit "underground" male lover than did women who were hospitalized for other reasons. McClelland (1963a) showed how this theme appeared consistently throughout popular Western literature and drama starting with Greece through the Middle Ages to the present in a form that he called the "Harlequin complex"—the name given in more recent times to the demon lover. Goleman (1976) found the theme in popular women's magazines in which a simple country girl is carried off by a dashing but dangerous man (sometimes a traveling salesman), only to discover he cannot be trusted. At that point in the Greek version of the myth, Medea deserts Jason with whom she has eloped, kills their children, and returns home. In the women's magazines, she turns her seducer over to the proper authorities and returns home to her boyhood lover. In the men's magazines, the story is told from the male point of view: Jason picks up a female companion to help him on his way to glory, only to find she betrays him and causes his downfall.

May (1980) developed TAT thematic coding systems to measure the rise and fall theme of Icarus and Jason and the fall and rise theme of Persephone and Medea. He called the former the enhancement–deprivation male theme and the latter, the deprivation–enhancement female theme; he found evidence that they were related to male and female sexuality (see McClelland, 1987). Building on earlier work by Beardslee and Fogelson (1958), Ouchida (1996) confirmed this connection indirectly. He checked an early hypothesis by Ellis (1954) that in the human species, change in the timbre of a male voice is the sign to a woman that a man is sexually mature. He found that women did produce more covert sexual imagery in TAT-type stories to music sung by male rather than female voices and that a male voice elicited more deprivation–enhancement female themes than a female voice in the women's stories. No differences in responses to gender of voice appeared in the men's stories, suggesting that the women were responding to male voices in a sexual way because the mature male voice signifies sexuality to women, as Ellis argued.

But McAdams most dramatically used the thematic potential of the TAT to develop a whole new approach to personality study. In *Power, Intimacy and the Life Story* (McAdams, 1985) and *Stories We Live by* (McAdams, 1993), he treated the life story that a person gradually creates over time as if it were a large and continuing TAT story. Then he analyzed it in terms of such themes as those just reviewed and many others often based on "imagoes" drawn from history or mythology. Thus, in prolonged interviews—which are really enlarged TATs—it may appear that a woman has created an image of herself as Hestia, the keeper of hearth and home in Greek mythology. The themes as they unfold over time account for much of what the person thinks, says, feels, and does. The TAT approach lives on here in a truly expanded narrative form.

Study of Cultural Themes

McClelland and Friedman (1952) recognized fairly early that popular literature, in this case folktales, might provide an insight into themes of a culture just as the TAT provides insight into themes in an individual's life. Applying TAT-type coding systems for motives or other variables to cultural, often historical documents opened up a whole new area of research, which has grown tremendously over the years. In an extension of the folktale study, it was found (McClelland, 1961) that high scores for n Achievement in the folktales of 52 preliterate tribes from around the world were associated with more active entrepreneurship in the culture, just as n Achievement was associated with entrepreneurship at the individual level. Then samples of Greek literature (including poems, epigrams, funeral orations, war speeches of encouragement, etc.) drawn by Berlew (1956, published in McClelland, 1958) comparable at three different historical periods were scored for n Achievement, showing that high levels of n Achievement preceded economic expansion and lower levels, economic decline—again a result that corresponds to a relationship at the individual level (McClelland & Franz, 1992). In later studies, researchers used such varied sources as sea captains' letters home, hymns, popular fiction, and stories for children sampled over long time periods to trace changes in historical levels of the three basic motives in English, Spanish, and U.S. history and the relationship of those changes to such variables as likelihood of going to war, levels of patent applications, or rates of economic growth (McClelland, 1987).

Stories from children's readers from the third to the fifth grade were assumed to be the simplest, most spontaneous expressions of cultural themes in a fashion paralleling the TAT. In any case, they proved to be a comparable and rich source of motive and thematic characteristics like other directedness, which across samples of countries predicted rates of economic growth, levels of investment in defense spending, and so forth (McClelland, 1961, 1975).

An analysis of speeches and other free verbal expressions, for example, in recorded interviews, enabled Winter and Stewart (1977), Zullow and Seligman (1990), and Peterson (1992) to look at motive levels, explanatory style, and other such variables that predict which politicians are likely to be elected and how they will behave after elected. Winter's (1996) analysis of Richard Nixon is a particularly interesting expansion of a TAT-type diagnosis of a public figure. It is reminiscent of the seminar Murray conducted in 1949–1950 analyzing the fantasies, interviews, and speeches of

Whittaker Chambers and others in an effort to clear Alger Hiss of Richard Nixon's accusation that he was a communist agent.

Cultural themes from children's stories have also been analyzed to diagnose characteristics of a culture or nation state in much the same way as material is used to diagnose an individual's personality. For example, I found several recurrent themes in stories drawn from children's readers of three major linguistic groups in India (McClelland, 1975). The stories stressed, for example, that merit is attained by giving, giving expresses power needs and implies a superior–subordinate relationship, and to give one must accumulate resources, which can lead to competition over resources. This thematic complex was used to account for some unique characteristics of Indian culture such as the use of fasting to attain political goals, the relative importance of women in politics, the naturally gifted having more resources, and the view of work as giving service rather than as getting something done.

In effect, I argued that the TAT-like quality of imaginative stories by children enables the observer to find key cultural themes, which account for the culture's unique characteristics, just as a similar analysis of a TAT permits an explanation of many of the key symptoms or unique traits of an individual (McClelland, 1975). The method has important applications for the study of culture at a distance from mythology, popular literature, and so on, that is much less labor intensive than national public opinion polls for explaining key characteristics of a culture. The method has not been adopted by cultural anthropologists or students of national character. Yet the studies carried out so far (see McClelland, 1975, on Mexico and a comparison of Turkey and Iran by McClelland, 1963b) suggest that the method is valid, so far as accounting for some unique characteristics of the nations involved is concerned.

The Behavioral Event Interview and the Study of Competence

In the early 1970s, the U.S. Navy was concerned about its poor race relations. It had responded to the challenge of trying to treat Blacks fairly and upgrading them according to appropriate standards of competence by creating officers who were in effect human relations consultants on racial matters, but the Navy did not seem to be very effective in reducing racial prejudice. So Navy representatives came to me and asked if I could make suggestions as to how their race relations consultants could be trained to do a better job. I replied that so far as I knew, little had been discovered on how to rid people of prejudice other than to assign them to work together on similar jobs—a finding that had come out of World War 2. So in the absence of knowledge, it seemed foolish to design a training course. Instead, what made sense was to find race relations consultants who were doing the job well and study carefully how they went about their job—for example, how they felt, thought, talked, and acted as compared with other consultants who were not doing very well with the same responsibilities.

The Navy agreed to fund the finding of an answer to this fundamental research question first.

In a way, the question was similar to the one Murray and his associates (Office of Strategic Services Assessment Staff, 1948) attempted to answer when they set up the Office of Strategic Services Research Program to find out how to create successful spies. But in my project, I did not follow their research plan that consisted of trying to figure out in advance how expert spies would think, talk, and act (e.g., by being able to maintain cover stories) and then of developing tests to check their hypotheses. Instead, I decided on a completely open-ended approach in which I designed an interview procedure modeled as closely as possible after the TAT. Here, I was influenced by what had happened in a seminar I attended on the TAT conducted by Murray. Everyone was asked to administer the TAT and to bring in the stories for analysis to the next session. One student complained that he had been unable to get his participant to tell any stories. They were short, thin, and not at all revealing. Murray responded by saying, "Let me have a try at it"; the next week, he brought in long, full, imaginative stories from the same participant. I learned that with Murray's somewhat hesitant yet curious and probing approach, one could get full-blown imaginative stories from anyone.

So I encouraged the interviewee—in this case, a race relations consultant—to recount in full detail six stories or episodes in his or her work life as a consultant: three stories around events that turned out well from his or her viewpoint and three that did not turn out well. The instructions for telling the stories were very similar to those for the TAT: Tell me what happened. How did the event start? Who was involved? What was thought? Who thought this? What was said? How did you feel? What was done? How did it turn out? Notice the emphasis was not, as in typical interviews, on what happened in the external world, usually as summarized, conceptualized, and editorialized by the interviewee. Instead, I wanted words said, feelings expressed, and so forth. The emphasis was on getting inside the head of the person telling the story, just as the TAT instructions are designed to do. In a sense, I almost did not care whether the stories people were telling were "really" true or accurate because what I cared about was whether they were a true report of thoughts, feelings, and actions of the person being interviewed.

By this method, I was able to distinguish how the outstanding consultants differed from the typical ones in any of a variety of possible ways. Then my task was to develop scoring systems for these differences, similar to the motive scoring systems developed for the TAT. In this case, I was able to code reliably seven different thematic characteristics that were shown significantly more often by the outstanding race relations consultants than the typical race relations consultants. These I called "competencies" because they were clearly related to being successful on the job. With the help of the Navy, a training program was then developed to teach consultants these competencies needed for the job (Spencer & Spencer, 1993).

The TAT-type interview was labeled the Behavioral Event Interview;

it has formed the basis of dozens of similar studies designed to determine the competencies associated with success in a variety of managerial or leadership positions. Gradually, a dictionary of competencies commonly found to differentiate outstanding from typical performers in a job was developed (Spencer & Spencer, 1993), which is not unlike the dictionary Murray (1938) developed to describe the various codes his group decided to use for personality. The chief differences are that the competency dictionary does not attempt to cover all aspects of personality but only competencies and that its codes are based on empirical rather than dictionary definitions.

A review of these competency studies (McClelland, 1997) building on an earlier one (Boyatzis, 1982) reveals that about 12 competencies have most often been associated with successful managerial performance across 64 cases. They include such characteristics as achievement orientation, analytical thinking, information seeking, interpersonal understanding, organizational awareness, impact and influence, and initiative in planning ahead. In different managerial positions in different organizations, different combinations of these core competencies are associated with success; but in nearly all cases, at least one individual initiative type and one organizational type competency is necessary for success. That is, a person must show either achievement orientation or initiative and either organizational know-how or impact and influence. Thus, there is no one cookie-cutter model of the successful executive in these jobs. Instead, people with somewhat different characteristics drawn from certain categories plus competencies unique to that organization are associated with success.

In the case of a particular position, the competencies that characterize outstanding performers (including the unique ones) are woven into an overall picture that describes how they fit together to lead to outstanding performance. A good example of such a competency model is for outstanding leadership of U.S. Catholic religious orders (Nygren & Ukeritis, 1993). It also illustrates the complete flexibility of finding new and important characteristics from the TAT-type open interview because one of the competencies that differentiated the outstanding from the typical religious leaders was frequent awareness of the presence of God—a characteristic that does not appear in Murray's dictionaries or in most psychologists' conceptualizations. This approach to identifying competencies on the basis of a TAT-type interview has proven to be of great usefulness to business organizations. In one company, for example (McClelland, 1997), it consistently identified the competencies associated with managerial success, provided a basis for feedback to executives to help them approach their jobs better, cut executive turnover thus saving far more money than the system cost, and provided a method of selecting new hires who would perform more successfully in the 1st year on the job.

Conclusion

Such an extension in the use of the TAT approach would have surprised Murray because it was far from his areas of interest. In addition, it would have provided him with further reason for teasing me about my obsession, as he saw it, for doing things efficiently and making money. He used to complain frequently that I would not talk to him often enough and used to offer, jokingly, to pay me for my time because money was what interested achievement-oriented people like me.

But for me, this is just one more indication of how powerful the idea behind the TAT is for creating new insights into human nature. What is basic to all these extensions of the TAT is the insistence that spontaneous, imaginative thought when analyzed for content can provide psychological information that goes far beyond what is obtained from self-edited conscious reports or from limited responses to particular stimuli as in stimulus–response psychology. Following this lead, I see a new interest in the psychology of mental content (McClelland, 1955) or a revolutionary shift from respondent to operant psychology (McClelland, 1984). Certainly following this lead has opened whole new avenues for contributions psychology can make to economics and business, history, political science and international relations, and cultural anthropology and sociology. It has even opened a new avenue to approach psychotherapy by leading to courses that have successfully changed personality characteristics, such as motives (McClelland & Winter, 1971) or competencies (Boyatzis, Cowen, Kolb, & Associates, 1995). Surely Murray and Morgan would be somewhat amazed to observe what has happened to their idea of creating a useful clinical instrument for diagnosing deep unconscious motives and complexes.

References

Allport, G. (1937). *Personality, a psychological interpretation*. New York: Holt.

Atkinson, J. W. (1958). Towards experimental analysis of human motivation in terms of motives, expectancies and incentives. In J. W. Atkinson (Ed.), *Studies in fantasy, action and society* (pp. 288–305). Princeton, NJ: Van Nostrand.

Atkinson, J. W., & McClelland, D. C. (1948). The effect of different intensities of the hunger drive on thematic apperception. *Journal of Experimental Psychology, 38*, 643–658.

Beardslee, D. C., & Fogelson, R. (1958). Sex differences in sexual imagery arousal by musical stimulation. In J. W. Atkinson (Ed.), *Studies in fantasy, action and society* (pp. 143–159). Princeton, NJ: Van Nostrand.

Berlew, D. E. (1956). *The achievement motive and the growth of Greek civilization*. Unpublished bachelor's thesis, Wesleyan University.

Boyatzis, R. E. (1982). *The competent manager: A model for effective performance*. New York: Wiley.

Boyatzis, R. E., Cowen, S. S., Kolb, D. A., & Associates. (1995). *Innovation in professional education*. San Francisco: Jossey-Bass.

Ellis, H. (1954). *The psychology of sex*. New York: New American Library.

Entwistle, D. R. (1972). To dispel fantasies about fantasy-based measures of achievement motivation. *Psychological Bulletin, 77*, 377–391.

Goleman, D. (1976, April). Jason and Medea's love story. *Psychology Today, 9*, 84–86.

May, R. (1980). *Sex and fantasy*. New York: Norton.

McAdams, D. P. (1985). *Power, intimacy and the life story*. New York: Guilford Press.

McAdams, D. P. (1993). *Stories we live by: Personal myths and the making of the self*. New York: Morrow.

McClelland, D. C. (1942). Functional autonomy of motives as an extinction phenomenon. *Psychological Review, 49,* 272–283.

McClelland, D. C. (1955). The psychology of mental content reconsidered. *Psychological Review, 62,* 297–302.

McClelland, D. C. (1958). The use of measures of human motivation in the study of society. In J. W. Atkinson (Ed.), *Motives in fantasy, action and society* (pp. 518–552). New York: Van Nostrand.

McClelland, D. C. (1961). *The achieving society.* New York: Van Nostrand.

McClelland, D. C. (1963a). The harlequin complex. In R. W. White (Ed.), *The study of lives* (pp. 94–120). New York: Atherton.

McClelland, D. C. (1963b). National character and economic growth in Turkey and Iran. In L. W. Pye (Ed.), *Communication and political development* (pp. 112–132). Princeton, NJ: Princeton University Press.

McClelland, D. C. (1975). *Power: The inner experience.* New York: Irvington.

McClelland, D. C. (1984). Motives as sources of long-term trends in life and health. In D. C. McClelland (Ed.), *Motives, personality and society: Selected papers* (pp. 343–364). New York: Praeger.

McClelland, D. C. (1987). *Human motivation.* New York: Cambridge University Press.

McClelland, D. C. (1989). Motivational factors in health and disease. *American Psychologist, 44,* 675–683.

McClelland, D. C. (1995). Achievement motivation in relation to achievement-related recall, performance and urine flow, a marker associated with release of vasopressin. *Motivation and Emotion, 19,* 59–76.

McClelland, D. C. (1997). *Use of behavioral interviews to assess competencies associated with executive success.* Unpublished manuscript, McBer, Boston, MA.

McClelland, D. C., Atkinson, J. W., Clark, R. A., & Lowell, E. L. (1953). *The achievement motive.* New York: Appleton-Century-Crofts.

McClelland, D. C., Davidson, R., Saron, C., & Floor, E. (1980). The need for power, brain norepinephrine turnover and learning. *Biological Psychology, 10,* 93–102.

McClelland, D. C., & Franz, C. E. (1992). Motivational and other sources of work accomplishment in mid-life: A longitudinal study. *Journal of Personality, 60,* 679–707.

McClelland, D. C., & Friedman, G. A. (1952). Child-rearing and the achievement motivation appearing in folktales. In G. E. Swanson, T. M. Newcomb, & E. L. Hartley (Eds.), *Readings in social psychology* (2nd ed., pp. 243–249). New York: Holt, Rinehart, & Winston.

McClelland, D. C., Koestner, R., & Weinberger, J. (1989). How do self-attributed and implicit motives differ? *Psychological Review, 96,* 690–702.

McClelland, D. C., Maddocks, J. A., & McAdams, D. P. (1985). The need for power, brain norepinephrine turnover and memory. *Motivation and Emotion, 9,* 1–10.

McClelland, D. C., Patel, V., Stier, D., & Brown, D. (1987). The relationship of affiliative arousal to dopamine release. *Motivation and Emotion, 11,* 51–66.

McClelland, D. C., & Pilon, D. A. (1983). Sources of adult motives in patterns of parent behavior in early childhood. *Journal of Personality and Social Psychology, 44,* 564–574.

McClelland, D. C., & Winter, D. G. (1971). *Motivating economic achievement.* New York: Free Press.

McGaugh, J. L. (1990). Significance and remembrance: The role of neuromodulatory systems. *Psychological Science, 1,* 15–25.

Murray, H. A. (Ed.). (1938). *Explorations in personality: A clinical and experimental study of fifty men of college age.* New York: Oxford University Press.

Nygren, D. J., & Ukeritis, M. (1993). *The future of religious orders in the United States: Transformation and commitment.* Westport, CT: Praeger.

Office of Strategic Services Assessment Staff. (1948). *Assessment of men.* New York: Rinehart.

Ouchida, M. (1996). *Gender differences in sexual imagery aroused by vocal music.* Unpublished master's thesis, Harvard University.

Peterson, C. (1992). Explanatory style. In C. P. Smith (Ed.), *Motivation and personality: Handbook of thematic content analysis* (pp. 376–382). New York: Cambridge University Press.

Robinson, F. G. (1992). *Love's story told: A life of Henry A. Murray.* Cambridge, MA: Harvard University Press.

Sanford, R. N. (1937). The effect of abstinence from food upon imaginal processes: A further experiment. *Journal of Psychology, 3,* 145–159.

Saudino, K., & Plomin, R. (1996). Personality and behavior genetics: Where have we been and where are we going? *Journal of Research in Personality, 30,* 335–347.

Smith, C. P. (Ed.). (1992). *Motivation and personality: Handbook of thematic content analysis.* New York: Cambridge University Press.

Spangler, W. D. (1992). Validity of questionnaire and TAT measures of need for achievement: Two meta-analyses. *Psychological Bulletin, 112,* 140–154.

Spencer, L. M., Jr., & Spencer, S. M. (1993). *Competence at work: Models for superior performance.* New York: Wiley.

Veroff, J., Depner C., Kulka, R., & Douvan, E. (1980). Comparison of American motives: 1957 versus 1976. *Journal of Personality and Social Psychology, 39,* 1249–1262.

Winter, D. G. (1973). *The power motive.* New York: Free Press.

Winter, D. G. (1996). *Personality: Analysis and interpretation of lives.* New York: McGraw-Hill.

Winter, D. G., & Stewart, A. J. (1977). Power motive reliability as a function of retest instructions. *Journal of Consulting and Clinical Psychology, 45,* 436–440.

Zullow, H. M., & Seligman, M. E. P. (1990). Pessimistic rumination predicts defeat in presidential candidates, 1900–1984. *Psychological Inquiry, 1,* 52–61.

14

Cross-Cultural–Multicultural Use of the Thematic Apperception Test

Richard H. Dana

My introduction to cross-cultural personality study began when I was a graduate student and was facilitated by Thematic Apperception Test (TAT) stories and Rorschach protocols from Chinese students (Dana, 1959a). I learned from this process that in using cross-cultural interpretation of projective techniques, one could not assume that the meanings of scores and inferences were invariant and universal; they were instead culture specific and could be understood only by an immersion in the culture. A dissatisfaction with psychiatric diagnoses of multicultural people led to my awareness that the TAT can provide information on the cultural self. This information is relevant for descriptions of cultural identity or cultural conflict and is necessary for the cultural formulations now required to increase the reliability and accuracy of a diagnosis using the *Diagnostic and Statistical Manual of Mental Disorders* (4th ed. [*DSM-IV*]; American Psychiatric Association, 1994).

In all of these ventures with the TAT cards, my former teacher, Silvan Tomkins's (1947) exquisite distillation of a methodology for examining the richness of a person has remained with me to guide my interpretations in reports that can be shared with assessees and subsequently amplified by their own self-understanding.

Historic Background

Cross-cultural use of the TAT began soon after the publication of the cards, providing pictorial stimuli for Henry Murray's need–press personality theory with scoring variables for needs and presses representing internal processes and external influences (Murray, 1938, 1943). The zeitgeist soon dictated that only needs would become a major focus for research. A literature developed that included very few needs but became a powerful demonstration of methodology and potential real-world applications for a projective test (for a review, see Dana, 1968). This literature, then and now, fails to capture the interest of most clinical psychologists, who prefer to interpret the TAT idiosyncratically in accordance with their own intuition. Other approaches to formal scoring systems for research or practice have been experienced by many as cumbersome, time consuming, and conceptually limited. Vane (1981) discovered only five of these systems with standardization data for Anglo Americans surviving in doctoral programs, including Murray's needs and my system for gross psychiatric screening (Brookings, 1995; Dana, 1959b)—two approaches that with some alterations now have applicability for multicultural populations.

Assessment practice with the TAT was nourished by a variety of early approaches to interpretation (e.g., Henry, 1956; Shneidman, 1951; Stein, 1955; Tomkins, 1947). Tomkins taught me that even brief TAT stories can be transformed by assessor fantasy into powerful and credible personality portraits. However, TAT training in doctoral programs has decreased dramatically over time (Piotrowski & Zalewski, 1993), and TAT usage has declined in general assessment practice (Piotrowski, Belter, & Keller, 1998) except with adolescents (Archer, Maruish, Imhof, & Piotrowski, 1991); in addition, optimism concerning TAT reliability and validity research has waned (Keiser & Prather, 1990), particularly among psychologists who demand a rigorous psychometric basis for assessment (Piotrowski & Keller, 1984; Polyson, Norris, & Ott, 1985).

These outcomes have occurred, I believe, for two reasons. First, there was an early debate concerning the necessity for any objective scoring whatsoever, and second, assessor fantasy was a poor substitute for scores derived from theory that could be applied reliably and their conceptual meaning subsequently validated.

In this chapter, I examine not only the continuing interest in TAT applications to multicultural populations but also briefly revisit hoary controversial issues, including card stimuli, scoring, interpretation, and research that affect usage with all populations. These discussions provide a context for examining the current status and future prospects for cross-cultural and multicultural TAT research and applications.

Many Tests or Just One?

By the mid-1940s, anthropologists and others began to alter the Murray cards by redrawing the originals for culture-specific populations or by designing and using different pictures (for a review, see Dana, 1993). Clearly delineated criteria were soon available for the design of new pictures (Sherwood, 1957). The use of many redrawn sets of TAT cards and the appearance of new picture-story tests diluted research interest in the further development of a standard scoring system for Murray's original TAT.

A carefully developed system can be reliably applied and validated for personality and psychopathology variables (see Abrams, chap. 12, this volume). The continued use of pictures with a known research history and a historic attention to collection of normative data still has merit as a context for interpretation (for a review, see Dana, 1982a). There are strong reasons as well to continue the unfinished clinical research with early scoring systems, particularly the Murray system that has only prospered in nonclinical research. This research is necessary for the development of a consensual scoring system, analogous to Herman Rorschach's original scores that remain largely intact with only embellishments and an accumulating research history.

Scoring Variables

First-generation clinical psychological wisdom provided guidelines for TAT interpretation distilled from accumulated experience with both the *physical* structure (what is present in the picture) and the *psychological* structure (interpretative value of each picture). Included were story characteristics, congruence with test stimuli, conformity with directions, conflict and distance indexes, and literal contents as well as rudimentary thematic norms (Dana, 1982a, 1996; Holt, 1978). These early guidelines, however, predated an empirical research literature, were applicable primarily to men of college age and older, and are now outdated. Moreover, the Anglo American emic source of these normative expectations also limits generalizability to multicultural people who are assimilated or bicultural in cultural orientation status.

Formal scoring variables can be developed from domains the TAT is known to assess, as first compiled by Shneidman (1951), for example, and supplemented by more recent research elaboration of particular scores. Moreover, for adolescents and children at least, these guidelines can be augmented by hypotheses with empirical origins. More specifically, existing scores may be used or new scores developed for affect quality, cognitions, control–defenses, conflict areas, ego strength, identity, needs, psychopathology, self-regulation, and sex role development (Dana, 1986; Teglasi, 1993). Because the TAT is used as a projective interview with a "doctrinaire integration of inferred psychoanalytic interpretation" (Rossini & Moretti, 1997, p. 395), the future of TAT usage in the United States will depend on a serious effort to develop a set of acceptable scoring categories that tap what the test can potentially measure (Dana, 1997). Normative data should be developed for these categories. Validation can be provided by the model described later in this chapter using reports rather than TAT scores. Additionally, the Murray TAT should be adapted for multicultural populations.

Many early scoring systems were developed for general use. Shneidman (1951; chap. 7, this volume) juxtaposed 16 methods of analysis— including normative, hero-oriented, intuitive, interpersonal, and perceptual approaches—to describe the potential information obtainable from a single set of TAT stories. The contents in these reports were abstracted and clustered into categories. The percentages of statements by categories follow: symptoms, diagnoses, and etiology (15.0%); personality defenses and mechanisms (12.0%); affect, feelings, and emotions other than hostility (10.0%); interpersonal and object relations–attitudes toward–from parents (9.0%); sexual thought and behavior (9.0%); outlook, attitudes, and beliefs (8.0%); quality of perception, fantasy, language, and thought (5.0%); frustrations, conflicts, and fears (5.0%); prognoses, predictions, and treatment (4.0%); motivations, goals, and drives (4.0%); reality contact and orientation (3.0%); interpersonal and object relations other than parents (3.0%); hostility (3.0%); intellect and abilities (2.0%); self-concept and insight into self (2.0%); self-control, ego strength, and ego capacity (2.0%); superego, values, and ego ideal (2.0%); postdictions of factual biographical data (2.0%) and psychological biographical data (1.0%); psychosexual level and development (0.2%); and pressures, forces, and presses (0.2%).

I listed these contents in their entirety to suggest that the TAT may not be so different from the Rorschach in the capacity to elicit personality and psychopathological materials when a similar method is used. For example, a factor analysis of clusters of concepts contained in 31 Rorschach reports by eight examiners included interpretive content for interpersonal relationships, disruptive internal processes, rigidity, intellectual control, achievement, creative imagination, timidity, affectional needs, self-concept, authority, inertia, and obsessive control (Dana, Bonge, & Stauffacher, 1981).

Validation Research

In the absence of consensual scoring permitting an accumulation of research findings over time, the usefulness of the TAT lacks adequate documentation for research-oriented generations of clinical psychologists. These psychologists prefer validating evidence or observable consequences rather than procedural evidence—a combination of consistency, intelligibility, and communal common sense (Rychlak, 1959). As a consequence, test scores are used as measures of concepts. Validating evidence is then related to external criteria to obtain concurrent or predictive validities. The hypothetical concepts undergirding the test scores are examined using construct validity by correlations with other tests, factor analysis, age differentiation, internal consistency, convergent and discriminant validation, and experimental interventions. Using this model, validity studies of projective tests include so many methodological errors that Anastasi (1982) concluded that these tests are poor vehicles to demonstrate the utility of the scientific method. Cross-cultural construct validation depends primarily on factor analysis because convergent–discriminant analysis and other approaches are much more difficult to apply. In fact, Shneidman (1959) once referred to construct validation as "similar to measuring a floating cloud with a rubber band in a high wind" (p. 261).

Rorschach- and TAT-validation studies conducted with my students and a subsequent review of cross-cultural construct validation literature (Dana, 1993) convinced me that a different validation paradigm is essential to demonstrate to increasingly skeptical and psychometrically informed professionals that these tests have continued clinical usefulness. For nearly 40 years, I have taught graduate students to learn projective technique interpretation by examining the validity of the concepts in their own reports. This method requires that a group of students and one or more experienced assessors use the same data for preparation of independent reports. The concepts in both student and criterion reports are then compared for agreements and disagreements. Using a minimum of four separate data sets, I found a consistent decrease in concept disagreements and a concomitant increase in agreements on concepts (Dana, 1982a). Student reports became indistinguishable in their contents from reports prepared by the more experienced assessors, although stylistic differences remained. As a byproduct of this method, my students also learned to separate their own fantasies and personality characteristics, or what I then called "eisegesis," from legitimate data-based inferences (Dana, 1966; Dana, Bolton, & West, 1983).

Competent TAT reports can provide the data for validation research because these reports delineate the personality and psychopathology content elicited from TAT protocols. Learning to prepare these TAT reports requires a set of formal scoring variables as well as the method to increase reliability by reducing the clinician's personalized fantasy contribution to reports.

Desiderata for Cross-Cultural–Multicultural Applications

The suggestions above for TAT scoring categories have Anglo American emic origins and require modification for multicultural populations in the United States. This is critical because Anglo American emics continue to be used as if they were etics when, in fact, they are pseudo-etics. Pseudo-etics have long been recognized as the most frequently used and least defensible methodological solution to the etic–emic dilemma or the difficulty in obtaining observations that are simultaneously both culturally adequate and cross-culturally comparable (Davidson, Jaccard, Triandis, Morales, & Diaz-Guerrero, 1976).

A second proposed solution is a combined approach in which an etic construct with apparent universal status is recognized. Emic measures of this construct are then constructed and validated independently in different cultures using the same methodology. This emic-ally defined etic construct is then used for cross-cultural comparisons. Diaz-Guerrero and Diaz-Loving (1990) argued coherently for cross-culturally validated etic or universal constructs that are found in the semantic differential technique, the State–Trait Anxiety Inventory, the Holtzman inkblot technique, the Embedded Figures Test, and the Rokeach Value Survey.

Several desiderata for cross-cultural picture-story tests have been suggested to minimize use of Anglo American emics as pseudo-etics (Dana, 1993).

1. The pictures should contain culturally recognizable figures in backgrounds designed to sample relevant interpretive domains, either by the selection of existing TAT cards to compose prototypical life situations (e.g., Dana, 1956) or by the redrawing of some or all of the original cards to more closely resemble the physical features of a particular cultural–racial population (e.g., Dana, 1982b). This goal can also be attained by a design of new pictures,

as in the Tell-Me-A-Story Test (see Costantino & Malgady, chap. 15, this volume).

2. Scoring variables developed in the United States should reflect characteristics that are culturally important in personality, psychopathology, culture-bound disorders, conditions due to oppression, and problems in living (Dana, 1998d). These scoring variables should also be independently developed and normed for each country in which the TAT is applied.

3. Normative data should be stratified by relevant moderator variables, such as educational level, social class, and acculturation status.

4. Information available within specific living environments should be used for documentation and verification of the scoring variables. This implies local consent, aegis, and direct participation, if not the actual development of scoring categories by local people.

5. Interpretation of these data should be made by reference to culture-specific personality theory and information on distressed or pathological behaviors of assessees.

Relevant personality information resources can be located, developed, and used in projective assessment training and practice with multicultural populations to increase cultural sensitivity, the reliability of inferences, and the accuracy of diagnostic statements (Dana, 1998c). This information is available in etic and emic social science research to a limited extent at this time. However, until this literature is more fully developed, emic contributions to literature constitute a major resource that often requires fluency in languages other than English. This information is mandatory for describing the cultural self in assessment for nonpsychiatric purposes and for contributing to the development of cultural formulations whenever a *DSM-IV* diagnosis is required.

Examples for Cross-Cultural Use

This section includes two examples for cross-cultural TAT use. An etic–emic approach uses Murray cards, an expanded set of "needs" or concerns, and a formal scoring system with a variety of populations on three continents. The second example, an emic approach, also uses Murray's original cards or those adapted for Plains Indians as well as generalized ostensibly pan-Indian, cross-cultural interpretive guidelines and psychological characteristics derived from exemplar TAT stories as a framework for TAT interpretation.

An Etic–Emic Approach

De Vos (1973) developed a psychocultural approach using Murray's cards noting 10 etic thematic concerns expressed as themes. These thematic concerns occur in human relations in one form or another, regardless of the cultural context, but are reported in emic normative data with major differences among these cultural groups. These concerns are instrumental or goal oriented (i.e., achievement, control, cooperation–competition, competence, and responsibility) and expressive (i.e., pleasure, nurturance, affiliation, appreciation, and harmony). In instrumental behavior–fantasy, "action is perceived by the self and others as motivated toward achieving a goal or meeting a standard by which behavior is judged" (De Vos, 1973, p. 35). Expressive behavior–fantasy consists of aroused feeling states.

In the words of David Ephraim (1997),

> the scoring system should be used heuristically, as a first attempt to describe the plot structures. The uniqueness of the narratives of a particular group, or the uniqueness of a particular narrative within a group, is as important as the features it shares with other stories. The meaning of a certain theme in a story may eventually be understood in the context provided by the rest of the stories of a cultural group.

Researchers have examined theme differences by card for various cultural groups and within-group social class distinctions, including Anglo Canadians, Venezuelans, Koreans, and Japanese Americans (e.g., Nisei and Issei; see DeVos, 1983; Ephraim, in press; and Ephraim, Sochting, & Marcia, 1997). In each of these cultural groups, for example, achievement motivation—an etic need—is displayed within either a person-centered or collectivist context and with an emic meaning linked to explicit goals, preferred means, and work-related beliefs (Dana, 1998a).

As this description suggests, these scoring procedures are both difficult to learn and time consuming to apply. Nonetheless, if these scoring categories do, in fact, represent a variety of basic or universal human concerns or genuine etics, the acquisition of emic normative data to indicate their relative importance across different cultural or national contexts becomes a legitimate and sorely needed research model. Moreover, any methodology for making etic comparisons across national groups using categories with emic norms may ultimately provide a model for TAT use with culturally diverse populations within the United States.

There is an immediate application of these research findings by practitioners who may currently use less formal procedures for interpretation in any of the countries in which the methodology has been applied. What to look for in story content from particular cards becomes more apparent as a result of labeling instrumental and expressive needs. However, if clinicians are to learn to reliably identify these concerns, representative national norms are needed. The scoring procedures themselves will then have to be taught to clinicians with the same care and time allocation that have gone into Rorschach training for generations. This is a relatively long-range research and training solution to an immediate practical need.

An Emic Approach

An exclusively emic approach is acceptable and applicable at this time for TAT assessment practice, particularly during a period when some assessors are insisting that culture-specific models of assessment–intervention are now both feasible and required (Dana, 1997, in press). The example chosen here is derived from data on only three American Indian tribes and is of unknown generalizability to other tribes, but the method can be replicated for other cultural groups in the United States. Either Murray's original cards are used or these cards are redrawn to include figures who resemble Indian people, and cards with scenes that represent unique or typical reservation settings and experiences are added (Dana, 1982b). This combination of cards increases the likelihood that culture-specific themes and content will be included in the stories. This approach combines two distinct parts: first, an examination and delineation of psychological characteristics reflected in TAT story structure and content and, second, a use of general guidelines for interpretation of projective techniques.

Monopoli (1984) developed 15 variables (also described in Dana, 1993), which were abstracted from archival Murray 20-card TAT protocols of previously identified traditional and acculturated Hopi, Zuni, and Navajos. These variables included economic deprivation–physical suffering, loneliness–isolation, interpersonal conflict–violence, individualistic versus familistic, time orientation, reactions to ambiguous stimuli, conception of experience, action sequence versus character development, views of nature, views of disease, morality, average story length, range of events–situations, alternative actions–choices–solutions by hero–heroine, and afterlife orientations.

The Indians' stories containing these variables were typically brief, literal, limited in contents to the reservation world, simply told, with hero and other characters of equal importance. Action sequences were central, unelaborated, and followed one after another with character development used only to advance the narrative. Abrupt organization shifts were frequent but were not interpreted as evidence for confusion or disorientation. Interpretive comments driven by projection were frequent, whereas intraceptive comments attributing characteristics to characters were rare. There was little differentiation between human and environmental details or between neutral and emotionally loaded events in stories in contrast to protocol content obtained from Anglo Americans.

A dampening of emotional experience in the stories can be associated with poverty, but the caveat here is that stereotypy is possible as well as association with a so-called "culture of poverty." Nonetheless, emotional restraint was also noted in another tribal setting with achromatic cards (Bigart, 1971), although it might not occur with chromatic cards (Johnson & Dana, 1965). The presence of an Anglo American examiner can also be responsible for restraint, control, and containment in TAT story content.

These TAT stories did not consist of themes, but instead a typical unfolding of picture details emerged gradually in mosaic fashion. Actions were motivated by outside events, and story characters were related by common family or community activities in lieu of interpersonal relationships, as is common among Anglo Americans. Generic identifications of people rather than relationships were used. Self-referents or internalized motivations were generally negative, and interpersonal tensions surfaced obliquely in actions.

These materials provide a set of emic expectations for structure and content of TAT stories and may be used together with projective assessment guidelines that recognize extreme intragroup differences not only in living contexts and life styles but also in worldview components. The components include the contents of the self, values, spirituality, and health–illness beliefs as well as perceptions of the assessor, assessment services, and service delivery style (Dana, 1995).

These guidelines contain three steps. First, use of the assessee's first language within a credible and acceptable social etiquette for TAT administration is desirable to avoid the formidable problems of translation or the presence of an interpreter. An assessee's second language may, however, frequently be used in the United States. This issue was discussed for the TAT protocols of Spanish–English bilinguals (Suarez, 1987). The use of a translator or interpreter when necessary for TAT stories has not received attention in the literature. Such translations into English for subsequent interpretation may sometimes be required, and guidelines should be prepared noting problems and providing suggestions for increasing accuracy and fidelity.

Second, an acculturation evaluation prior to the administration of the TAT provides cultural orientation status information that becomes part of a cultural identity description. In addition to these independent information sources, it is helpful to use the TAT to describe the contents and priorities of a cultural self as an internal force field (Dana, in press).

Within this field of forces, the permeability of boundaries, particular contents included, and relative importance or magnitude of specific contents varies as a function of culture. For example, an American Indian–Alaskan Native self typically has permeable or fluid boundaries that encompass an extended family as well as the tribe and native community. In addition, for traditional, bicultural, and marginal people, plants, animals, and places may be augmented by supernatural and spiritual forces. In the extreme case of an indigenous healer, these components and the tribe–community may occupy most of the space in the presence of very permeable boundaries (for Rorschach example, see Dana, 1993). By contrast, a modal Anglo American self displays fixed, relatively rigid, and impermeable boundaries of the individual plus some tangible possessions and intangibles of control and power (Dana, 1998c). Given these differences in self from an Anglo American modal standard, American Indians–Alaskan Natives are frequently pathologized, and culture-specific or emic assessment and intervention procedures are frequently required (Dana, 1998d, in press).

A map of the cultural self is an identity portrait prepared during assessment. To the best of my knowledge, the TAT has not been used for this purpose, although there is one published example of a TAT Card 1 interpretation from an objective relations stance in which Schectman (1993) examined the self as mediator of experience and author of action. All of this cultural information subsequently informs any cultural formulation used to increase reliability and accuracy of psychiatric diagnosis, particularly to recognize culture-bound disorders. In the United States, a cultural formulation is now a mandatory assessment accompaniment of any *DSM-IV* diagnosis with multicultural populations (Dana, 1998b, 1998d).

Third, an interpretation process relies on clinical inference and formal scoring. The clinical inference process provides an opportunity to use all of the cultural identity information either for therapeutic assessment or for planning subsequent interventions. This is in addition to or separate from a cultural formulation used for diagnostic purposes. As indicated earlier, the absence of consensually acceptable formal scoring for the TAT, analogous to the Rorschach, has restricted the clinical usefulness of the TAT. Cross-cultural, emic applications do not necessarily immediately require formal scores and normative data (Herzberg, in press), although these interpretation resources must become available to sustain global assessment practice using the TAT during the next century.

Comparison of Etic–Emic and Emic Approaches

Earlier in this chapter, desiderata including culturally recognizable pictures, scoring variables germane to the culture, availability of normative data, and culture-specific interpretation procedures for these TAT applications were described. It is now feasible to compare the two approaches on these desiderata.

The etic–emic approach uses Murray's cards that are presumed to contain recognizable figures and settings yielding stories in various cultural and national settings. These etic scoring variables have been applied in a variety of national–cultural settings and are believed to be universal. Local normative data is required in each of these settings, and interpretation is setting specific and incorporates culture-specific contents.

The emic approach can use either the original Murray cards or preferably redrawings of the originals with the addition of new cards to ensure identification with characters and settings. The scoring variables immediately reflect the culture because they are derived from content and structure of local TAT stories rather than being pseudo-etics from Anglo American sources. Normative data, however, are lacking and need to be developed from a representative collection of TAT stories across traditional and acculturated reservation-based tribes and urban Indians. Such data would not only provide cross-validation of the scoring variables but also evidence changes over time since the original archival sources were collected. An interpretation of findings for American Indians–Alaskan Natives has to be local at first because of the variety of their cultural and linguistic origins, although there is some consensus that a core of pan-Indian cultural characteristics exists.

However, personality information is not readily available to inform

TAT interpretation, nor can the writing of Anglo anthropologists and ethnographers be accepted uncritically. Because this approach requires substantial clinical judgment and extrapolation from many sources of information, immersion in local culture and specific interpretation training is mandatory. Such training should, I believe, entail comparisons of concepts in reports between neophyte and experienced TAT assessors who have origins similar to assessees.

Conclusion

These two approaches or models, etic–emic and emic, represent the TAT literature on culturally diverse populations. There are TAT studies from many countries throughout the world. These reports reflect useful descriptions of personality in culture, clinical case studies, examinations of specific hypotheses, and attempts to provide interpretation from a pseudo-etic psychoanalytic perspective. However, these illustrative studies compose only an interesting mosaic, providing glimpses of people who are not Anglo

Exhibit 14.1. Development of Cross-Cultural Standards for Thematic Apperception Test Interpretation in Training, Research, and Practice

---

Step 1. *Libraries.* Develop Thematic Apperception Test (TAT) archival protocol libraries for training, research, and practice.

Step 2. *Training.* Students–practitioners learn interpretation by receiving feedback on the concepts present in their own reports. Feedback occurs by comparison of these concepts with criterion report contents prepared by culturally competent assessors and by acceptance or rejection of their concepts by assessees. Training materials include what the TAT can measure, how to make inferences, and where to locate sources of information to inform cross-cultural and multicultural practice. The training focuses on writing reports that provide information on cultural identity, delineation of the self, and cultural formulations.

Step 3. *Research.* Develop a research agenda from archival library collections by (a) updating normative data by group, (b) reexamining card hypotheses by groups, (c) systematically examining available scoring variables, (d) selecting existing bimodal moderator variables for routine use to evaluate acculturation (i.e., cultural orientation status), socioeconomic status, age, and gender.

Step 4. *Practice.* As a basis for TAT assessment practice, reports should rely on moderator data for cultural identity, scoring categories validated on cross-cultural and multicultural populations, and relevant normative data.

Step 5. *Resource Development.* Narrative psychologists have focused on storytelling to examine identity as contained in life stories that embody cultural roles and worldviews (e.g., Howard, 1991; McGill, 1992). This parallel area can inform TAT assessment with core cultural metaphors and themes that have been used in clinical practice with multicultural families. Narrative psychology also provides an independent source of cultural knowledge, particularly for therapeutic assessment (Shapiro, 1998).

Americans because there has been little empirical collection of normative data (e.g., Avila-Espada, in press; Zhang, Xu, Cai, & Chen, 1993).

Thus far in this chapter, I suggested an interface of familiar TAT issues, historic and contemporary, with problems of application to culturally diverse populations in the United States and elsewhere. Psychologists have some knowledge of what the TAT can divulge in personality description and diagnosis of psychological distress in the United States primarily with Anglo Americans. Nonetheless, the TAT is capable of being much more than an emic if an implementable cross-cultural validation process is forthcoming.

Consensual formal scoring may be unnecessary at the onset if the concepts in TAT reports can be used as a reliable and potentially researchable data set for training, research, and practice. I would suggest that psychologists now require emic libraries of TAT protocols for training, research, and practice. These protocol libraries should be culture specific and acquire representative TATs using Murray's cards or redrawn cards from acculturated and traditional populations in the United States as a basis for this research. Independent reports can be subsequently generated from these data sets by assessors differing in clinical skills and cultural competence. There can then be comparisons with criterion information on these assessees. The cultural contents of these protocol interpretations in the form of concepts generated by the most experienced and culturally competent assessors can provide culture-specific standards for TAT usefulness. Exhibit 14.1 suggests a general format for this process.

References

American Psychiatric Association. (1994). *Diagnostic and statistical manual of mental disorders* (4th ed.). Washington, DC: Author.

Anastasi, A. (1982). *Psychological testing.* New York: Macmillan.

Archer, R. P., Maruish, M., Imhof, E. A., & Piotrowski, C. (1991). Psychological test usage with adolescent clients: 1990 survey findings. *Professional Psychology: Research and Practice, 22,* 247–252.

Avila-Espada, A. (in press). Objective scoring for the TAT. In R. H. Dana (Ed.), *Handbook of cross-cultural and multicultural personality assessment.* Hillside, NJ: Erlbaum.

Bigart, J. R. (1971). Patterns of cultural change in a Salish Flathead community. *Human Organization, 30,* 229–237.

Brookings, J. B. (1995). "Objective" scoring of projective tests: A laboratory exercise using the Thematic Apperception Test (TAT). *Measurement Forum, 1*(1), 2–3.

Dana, R. H. (1956). Selection of abbreviated TAT sets. *Journal of Clinical Psychology, 12,* 36–40.

Dana, R. H. (1959a). American culture and Chinese personality. *Psychological Newsletter, 12,* 36–40.

Dana, R. H. (1959b). Proposal for objective scoring of the TAT. *Perceptual and Motor Skills, 11*(Suppl. 1), 27–43.

Dana, R. H. (1966). Eisegesis and assessment. *Journal of Projective Techniques and Personality Assessment, 30,* 215–222.

Dana, R. H. (1968). Thematic techniques and clinical practice. *Journal of Projective Techniques and Personality Assessment, 32,* 204–214.

Dana, R. H. (1982a). *A human science model for personality assessment with projective techniques.* Springfield, IL: Charles C Thomas.

Dana, R. H. (1982b). *Picture-story cards for Sioux/Plains Indians.* Fayetteville: University of Arkansas.

Dana, R. H. (1986). Thematic Apperception Test used with adolescents. In A. I. Rabin (Ed.), *Projective techniques for children and adolescents* (pp. 14–36). New York: Springer.

Dana, R. H. (1993). *Multicultural assessment perspectives for professional psychology.* Boston, MA: Allyn & Bacon.

Dana, R. H. (1995). Orientaciones para la evaluación de Hispanos en los Estados Unidos de Nortéamerica utilizando la prueba de Rorschach y el Test de Apercepión Temática [Guidelines for assessment of Hispanics in the United States using the Rorschach and Thematic Apperception Tests]. *Revista de la Sociedad Espanola del Rorschach y Metodos Proyectivos, 8,* 176–187.

Dana, R. H. (1996). The Thematic Apperception Test (TAT). In C. Newmark (Ed.), *Major psychological assessment instruments* (2nd ed., pp. 166–205). Boston: Allyn & Bacon.

Dana, R. H. (1997, September). Thematic apperception testing with children and adolescents in multicultural populations. In R. Dana (Chair), *Projective techniques with children and adolescents.* Symposium conducted at the 4th European Conference on Psychological Assessment, Lisbon, Portugal.

Dana, R. H. (1998a, August). The cultural context of TAT achievement motivation: A methodology and examples from Card 1. In G. Costantino (Chair), *Multicultural/cross-cultural motivation as assessed by the TAT and TEMAS.* Symposium presented at the 106th Annual Convention of the American Psychological Association, San Francisco.

Dana, R. H. (1998b). Cultural identity assessment of culturally diverse groups: 1997. *Journal of Personality Assessment, 70,* 1–16.

Dana, R. H. (1998c). Personality assessment and the cultural self: Emic and etic contexts as learning resources. In L. Handler & M. Hilsenroth (Eds.), *Teaching and learning personality assessment* (pp. 325–345). Hillsdale, NJ: Erlbaum.

Dana, R. H. (1998d). *Understanding cultural identity in intervention and assessment.* Thousand Oaks, CA: Sage.

Dana, R. H. (in press). The cultural self as a locus for assessment and intervention with American Indians/Alaska Natives. *Journal of Multicultural Counseling and Development.*

Dana, R. H., Bolton, B., & West, V. (1983). Validation of eisegesis concepts in assessment reports using the 16PF: A training method with examples. In S. Krug (Ed.), *Third International 16PF Conference Proceedings* (pp. 20–29). Champaign, IL: Institute for Personality and Ability Testing.

Dana, R. H., Bonge, D., & Stauffacher, R. (1981). Personality dimensions in Rorschach reports: An empirical synthesis. *Perceptual and Motor Skills, 52,* 711–715.

Davidson, A. R., Jaccard, J. J., Triandis, H. C., Morales, M. L., & Diaz-Guerrero, R. (1976). Cross-cultural model testing: Toward a solution of the emic–emic dilemma. *International Journal of Psychology, 11,* 1–13.

De Vos, G. A. (1973). *Socialization for achievement: Essays on the cultural psychology of the Japanese.* Berkeley: University of California Press.

De Vos, G. A. (1983). Achievement motivation and intra-family attitudes in immigrant Koreans. *Journal of Psychoanalytic Anthropology, 6,* 125–162.

Diaz-Guerrero, R., & Diaz-Loving, R. (1990). Interpretation in cross-cultural personality assessment. In C. R. Reynolds & R. W. Kamphaus (Eds.), *Handbook of psychological and educational assessment of children: Personality, behavior, and context* (pp. 491–523). New York: Guilford Press.

Ephraim, D. (1997, March). Psychocultural approach to TAT narratives: Multicultural practice applications. In R. H. Dana (Chair), *Personality assessment practice with multicultural populations.* Symposium conducted at the Society of Personality Assessment meeting, San Diego, CA.

Ephraim, D. (in press). Psychocultural approach to TAT scoring and interpretation. In R. H. Dana (Ed.), *Handbook of cross-cultural and multicultural personality assessment.* Hillsdale, NJ: Erlbaum.

Ephraim, D., Sochting, I., & Marcia, J. E. (1997). Cultural norms for TAT narratives in psychological practice and research: Illustrative studies. *Rorschachiana, 22,* 13–37.

Henry, W. E. (1956). *The analysis of fantasy: The Thematic Apperception Test in the study of personality.* New York: Wiley.

Herzberg, E. (in press). The utilization of TAT in multicultural societies: Brazil and the United States. In R. H. Dana (Ed.), *Handbook of cross-cultural and multicultural personality assessment.* Hillsdale, NJ: Erlbaum.

Holt, R. R. (Ed.). (1978). *Methods in clinical psychology. Vol. 1: Projective assessment.* New York: Plenum Press.

Howard, G. S. (1991). Culture tales: A narrative approach to thinking, cross-cultural psychology, and psychotherapy. *American Psychologist, 46,* 187–197.

Johnson, A. W., Jr., & Dana, R. H. (1965). Color on the TAT. *Journal of Projective Techniques and Personality Assessment, 29,* 178–182.

Keiser, R. E., & Prather, E. N. (1990). What is the TAT? A review of ten years of research. *Journal of Personality Assessment, 55,* 800–803.

McGill, D. W. (1992). The cultural story in multicultural family therapy. *Families in Society: The Journal of Contemporary Human Services, 73,* 339–349.

Monopoli, J. (1984). *A culture-specific interpretation of thematic test protocols for American Indians.* Unpublished master's thesis, University of Arkansas—Fayetteville.

Murray, H. A. (Ed.). (1938). *Explorations in personality: A clinical and experimental study of fifty men of college age.* New York: Oxford University Press.

Murray, H. A. (1943). *The Thematic Apperception Test: Manual.* Cambridge, MA: Harvard University Press.

Piotrowski, C., Belter, R. W., & Keller, J. W. (1998). The impact of "managed care" on the practice of psychological testing: Preliminary findings. *Journal of Personality Assessment, 70,* 441–447.

Piotrowski, C., & Keller, J. W. (1984). Attitudes toward clinical assessment by members of the AABT. *Psychological Reports, 55,* 831–838.

Piotrowski, C., & Zalewski, C. (1993). Training in psychodiagnostic testing in APA-approved PsyD and PhD clinical psychology programs. *Journal of Personality Assessment, 61,* 394–405.

Polyson, J., Norris, D., & Ott, E. (1985). The recent decline in TAT research. *Professional Psychology: Research and Practice, 16,* 26–28.

Rossini, E. D., & Moretti, R. J. (1997). Thematic Apperception Test (TAT) interpretation: Practice recommendations from a survey of clinical psychology doctoral programs accredited by the American Psychological Association. *Professional Psychology: Research and Practice, 28,* 393–398.

Rychlak, J. F. (1959). Clinical psychology and the nature of evidence. *American Psychologist, 11,* 642–648.

Schectman, F. (1993). The sense of self as seen on the Thematic Apperception Test: A case example. *British Journal of Projective Psychology, 38*(2), 31–36.

Shapiro, E. R. (1998). The healing power of culture stories: What writers can teach psychotherapists. *Cultural Diversity and Mental Health, 4,* 91–101.

Sherwood, E. T. (1957). On the designing of TAT pictures, with special reference to a set for an African people assimilating Western culture. *Journal of Social Psychology, 45,* 161–190.

Shneidman, E. S. (Ed.). (1951). *Thematic Apperception Test analysis.* New York: Grune & Stratton.

Shneidman, E. S. (1959). Suggestions for the delineation of validation studies. *Journal of Projective Techniques, 23,* 259–263.

Stein, M. I. (1955). *The Thematic Apperception Test: An introductory manual for its clinical use with adults.* Cambridge, MA: Addison-Wesley.

Suarez, M. G. (1987, August–September). *Implications of Spanish–English bilingualism on the TAT stories.* Paper presented at the 95th Annual Convention of the American Psychological Association, New York.

Teglasi, H. (1993). *Clinical use of story telling emphasizing the TAT with children and adolescents.* Boston: Allyn & Bacon.

Tomkins, S. S. (1947). *The Thematic Apperception Test.* New York: Grune & Stratton.

Vane, J. R. (1981). The Thematic Apperception Test: A review. *Clinical Psychology Review, 1,* 319–336.

Zhang, T., Xu, S., Cai, Z., & Chen, Z. (1993). Research on the Thematic Apperception Test: Chinese revision and its norms. *Acta Psychologica Sinica, 25,* 314–323.

15

The Tell-Me-A-Story Test: A Multicultural Offspring of the Thematic Apperception Test

Giuseppe Costantino and Robert G. Malgady

The Tell-Me-A-Story Test (TEMAS) is an offspring of the Thematic Apperception Test (TAT) technique (Murray, 1943) and was designed as a multicultural projective test for use with minority and nonminority children. The TEMAS was developed for Hispanic children and adolescents and later was expanded to include Blacks and Whites. Pilot studies are in progress assessing the validity of the Asian American version of the TEMAS, presenting Asian characters interacting in Asian American urban settings.

Unlike the traditional TAT, the TEMAS presents multicultural characters in urban settings. These characters are pictured engaging in antithetical situations representing interpersonal and intrapersonal conflicts. Thus, the TEMAS is an attempt to increase the ethnocultural relevance of projective stimuli to minority as well as nonminority children and to present familiar scenes associated with life experiences in urban settings. In this chapter, we discuss the development and use of the TEMAS.

Background: Projective Tests

Thematic apperception techniques and other traditional projective tests are based on the psychodynamic assumption that an individual projects onto ambiguous stimuli unconscious drives that are ordinarily repressed (Murray, 1951; Murstein, 1963). Early clinicians tended to place strong emphasis on the content analysis of TAT stories to understand personality dynamics. However, with the advent of ego psychology, clinicians began to refocus their attention from the content of the id to the structure of the ego. Ego psychology posited that whereas the id provided the energy to motivate behavior, ego structure was responsible for the nature and di-

We thank Juanita Goico and Erminia Costantino for the typing and technical assistance. Parts of this chapter are adapted from *TEMAS (Tell-Me-A-Story) Manual*, by G. Costantino, R. Malgady, and L. Rogler, 1988, Los Angeles, CA: Western Psychological Services. Copyright 1988 by Western Psychological Services. Adapted with permission.

rection of behavior. Consequently, there was a parallel shift in the analysis of TAT stories. The new emphasis focused primarily on the structure of the theme (how the story was told) and secondarily on the symbolic content of the story (what was told; Bellak, 1954).

The highly cognitive nature of TAT stories was recognized in the early 1960s. Holt (1960a, 1960b), for example, argued that TAT stories are not fantasies or products of primary processes but products of conscious cognitive processes. Although he labeled TAT productions "fantasies," Kagan (1956) emphasized the importance of analyzing the ego defenses of the stories in addition to their symbolic content. Even earlier, Bellak (1954) pointed out that TAT stories need to be analyzed for both content and structure.

The emphasis on cognitive processes in projective testing was the natural progression of the theoretical development of behaviorism, which converged into the cognitive theories of the 1970s. There has been an impetus among some cognitive–behavioral psychologists to integrate the basic assumptions of ego psychology and cognitive psychology in the application of projective analyses (M. P. Anderson, 1981; Bellak, 1954, 1989; Forgus & Shulman, 1979; Singer & Pope, 1978; Sobel, 1981). Interest in projective tests has been growing dramatically, even among cognitive psychologists. In fact, Sobel proposed the development of a "projective-cognitive" instrument to assess an individual's problem-solving strategies, coping skills, and self-instructional styles.

Traditionally in clinicians' analyses of responses to projective personality tests, Hispanic and Black children have been evaluated as less verbally fluent, less behaviorally mature, and more psychopathological than their nonminority counterparts (Ames & August, 1966; Booth, 1966; Costantino & Malgady, 1995; Dana, 1993; Durret & Kim, 1973). This is a particular problem because it has been widely acknowledged that the validity of projective techniques is impugned when administered to examinees that are verbally inarticulate (H. Anderson & Anderson, 1955; Reuman, Alvin, & Veroff, 1983). In contrast, minority children are articulate when tested with culturally sensitive instruments (Bailey & Green, 1977; Costantino & Malgady, 1983; Costantino, Malgady, & Vazquez, 1981; Malgady, 1996; Thompson, 1949).

Nonetheless, projective tests have not fared equally well, even with White children. Urging the development of new valid instruments, Gallager (1979) lamented that "we often curse the quality of the tools we have. But we are trapped by them" (p. 998). The literature also emphasizes the need to develop psychological tests for reliable and valid diagnosis and personality assessment of minority children (Padilla, 1979) and to create culture-specific norms for projective tests (Dana, 1986, and chap. 14, this volume; Exner & Weiner, 1982).[1]

---

[1]In testing culturally, linguistically, and ethnically–racially diverse children, examiners should be fluent in the language in which the examinees are dominant and should be familiar with the cultural ethnic–racial heritage of the children being tested (American Psychological Association, 1993; Costantino, Malgady, & Rogler, 1988; Dana, chap. 14, this volume).

Overview of the Tell-Me-A-Story Test

Based on these considerations, the TEMAS (in Spanish, meaning *themes*) was developed as a multicultural thematic apperception test for use with Puerto Rican, other Hispanic, Black, and White children. There are two basic similarities between the TAT and the TEMAS: Both are based on the constructs of *projection* (verbalizations in the form of genotypical motives in the narrative; Atkinson, 1981) and *identification* (of the examinee with the character in the story). The TEMAS is different from the TAT in that it was specifically developed for use with children and adolescents, and it has two parallel sets of stimulus cards, one set for minorities and the other for nonminorities. The TEMAS, therefore, has extensive normative data for both minorities and nonminorities. Unlike the TAT, which is frequently interpreted subjectively, the TEMAS is objectively scored by consensus for cognitive as well as affective and personality functions, and examinee profiles are developed based on T scores, percentage scores, and multicultural norms. The TEMAS stimulus cards diminish ambiguity so as to elicit specific responses and are in color, which has been found to facilitate verbalization and projection of emotional states.

Whereas the TAT focuses on intrapsychic dynamics, the TEMAS focuses on personality functions as manifested in interpersonal relationships and as internalized by the child. The TEMAS stimuli represent the polarities of negative and positive emotions, cognitions, and interpersonal functions. For example, adaptive and maladaptive interpersonal relationships are defined by the child's ability to synthesize the polarities of dependence–individuation, respect–disrespect, and nurturance–rejection, as reflected by their stories. The TAT stimuli are more heavily weighted to represent hostility, negative emotions, and depressive moods. The TAT uses the concept of ambiguous stimuli to elicit meaningful stories, whereas the TEMAS uses the concept of bipolar personality functions to elicit conflict resolution in the narrative.

Theoretical Framework

The principal rationale for the development of the TEMAS was the acknowledged need for a psychometrically sound multicultural TAT designed specifically for use with children and adolescents. It can be used normatively with children and adolescents from ages 5 to 13 years and used clinically with children and adolescents from ages 5 to 18 years.

The theory underlying the TEMAS incorporates a dynamic-cognitive framework, which states that personality development occurs within a psychocultural system. Within this system, individuals internalize the cultural values and beliefs of family and society (Bandura & Walters, 1967). Personality functions are learned initially through modeling (Bandura, 1977) and are then developed through verbal and imaginal processes (Paivio, 1971; Piaget & Inhelder, 1971). When a test's projective stimuli are similar to the circumstances in which the personality functions were originally learned, these functions are readily transferred to the testing situation and are projected into the thematic stories (Auld, 1954). Moreover, personality is a structure comprised of a constellation of motives, which are learned and internalized dispositions and interact with environmental stimuli to determine overt behavior in specific situations. Because these dispositions are not directly observable in clinical evaluation, projective techniques prove to be useful instruments in probing beneath the overt structure (*phenotype*) of the personality, thereby arousing the latent motives imbedded in the personality genotype. Hence, it is assumed that projective tests assess relatively stable individual differences in the strength of underlying motives that are expressed in narrative or storytelling. Atkinson (1981) emphasized that the analysis of narrative (thematic content) has a more solid theoretical foundation than ever before and "remains the most important and virtually untapped resource we have for developing our understanding of the behavior of an animal distinguished by its unique competence in language and use of symbols" (p. 126).

Stimulus Cards

Costantino (1978) created the settings, characters, and themes; Phil Jacobs, an artist who worked closely with Costantino, rendered the artwork. Over 100 pictures were drawn before the 23 standardized pictures were selected. The TEMAS cards are described in Exhibit 15.1.

There are two parallel versions of TEMAS pictures: The minority version consists of pictures featuring predominantly Hispanic and Black characters in an urban environment, and the nonminority version consists of corresponding pictures showing predominantly White characters in an urban environment. The various personality functions depicted in the two parallel sets of pictures present identical themes.

Both the minority and nonminority versions have a short form of 9 cards from the 23-card long form. Of the 9 short form cards, 4 are administered to both sexes and 5 are sex specific. Of the 23 long form cards, 12 are for both sexes, 11 are sex specific, and 1 is age specific. Furthermore, there are 4 cards with pluralistic characters, which can be used interchangeably for both the minority and nonminority versions.

Scoring

TEMAS protocols are scored on a detailed record booklet. Each story is scored separately for cognitive, affective, and personality functions, as shown in Exhibit 15.2. The 18 cognitive functions are scored in the following way. Reaction time is scored in seconds; total time in minutes and seconds. Fluency is indicated by the number of words per story. Conflict is scored *1* if it is not recognized and blank if it is recognized. Sequencing is scored *1* if it is omitted and blank if it is recognized. Imagination is scored *1* if the narrative is stimulus bound and blank if it abstracts beyond

Exhibit 15.1.   Picture Descriptions

The short administration form consists of 9 cards marked by an *. The long form consists of 23 cards.

Card 1 B:* A mother is giving a command to her son. A father is in the background. Friends are urging the boy to play basketball with them (designed to pull for the personality functions of interpersonal relations and delay of gratification).

Card 1 G:* A mother is giving a command to her daughter. A father is in the background. Friends are urging the girl to play basketball with them (designed to pull for the personality functions of interpersonal relations and delay of gratification).

Card 2: A father is watching television and drinking. A son and a daughter are standing beside him. A mother is seen carrying a baby and vacuuming. Another daughter and son are seen at the mother's side (designed to pull for interpersonal relations and moral judgment).

Card 3: A father is telling his son to do his homework. A mother is holding a plate and getting a glass. A daughter is doing her homework at the kitchen table. Another daughter and son are watching television (designed to pull for interpersonal relations, achievement motivation, and delay of gratification).

Card 4: An angry father is threatening the mother. The two sons and two daughters are standing by the mother. A girl lies in a bed with her face covered (designed to pull for interpersonal relations, aggression, anxiety/depression, and moral judgment).

Card 5: A youngster is sleeping in a bed dreaming of a picnic with a woman. A figure enters through the bedroom window at night (designed to pull for interpersonal relations and aggression).

Card 6: A boy and a girl dress up in grown-up clothes in the attic while looking nostalgically at a crib and some baby toys (designed to pull for interpersonal relations and sexual identity).

Card 7:* An angry mother is watching her son and daughter argue over a broken lamp (designed to pull for interpersonal relations, aggression, and moral judgment).

Card 8: A male teacher is reading to a class of attentive students. A female teacher or principal is showing a broken window to a mother and father with their son and daughter (designed to pull for interpersonal relations, aggression, achievement motivation, and moral judgment).

Card 9 B: A boy with outstretched arms is standing at the crossroads in a forest. Friends call him to join them for a walk on the right-hand road (designed to pull for interpersonal relations and anxiety/depression).

Card 9 G: A girl with outstretched arms is standing at the crossroads in a forest. Friends call her to join them for a walk on the right-hand road (designed to pull for interpersonal relations and anxiety/depression).

Card 10 B: A boy is standing in front of a piggy bank holding money while imagining himself looking at a bicycle in a shop window and buying an ice cream cone (designed to pull for delay of gratification).

Card 10 G: A girl is standing in front of a piggy bank holding money while imagining herself looking at a bicycle in a shop window and buying an ice cream cone (designed to pull for delay of gratification).

Exhibit continues

Exhibit 15.1.   (*Continued*)

Card 11: A woman is carrying grocery bags with a boy and girl helping her. A woman is trying to protect herself from two boys and a girl who are stealing groceries from her bags (designed to pull for interpersonal relations, aggression, and moral judgment).

Card 12 G: A group of four girls is fighting (designed to pull for interpersonal relations, aggression, and moral judgment).

Card 13 B: A boy is standing in front of a bathroom mirror imagining the reflection of his parents in the mirror (designed to pull for interpersonal relations self-concept and sexual identity).

Card 13 G: A girl is standing in front of a bathroom mirror imagining the reflection of her parents in the mirror (designed to pull for interpersonal relations self-concept and sexual identity).

Card 14 B*: A boy is studying in his room. A group of boys and girls is listening to music in the living room (designed to pull for interpersonal relations, achievement motivation, and delay of gratification).

Card 14 G*: A boy is studying in his room. A group of boys and girls is listening to music in the living room (designed to pull for interpersonal relations, achievement motivation, and delay of gratification).

Card 15* (minority version): A coach is giving an award to a group of baseball players. A policeman is arresting a group of three boys and one girl who have broken a window and stolen merchandise (designed to pull for interpersonal relations, aggression, achievement motivation, and moral judgment).

Card 15* (nonminority version): A coach is giving an award to a group of soccer players. A policeman is arresting a group of three boys and one girl who have broken a window and stolen merchandise (designed to pull for interpersonal relations, aggression, achievement motivation, and moral judgment).

Card 16: A boy is climbing up a rope in gym, where a girl is jumping over a wooden horse. A group of two boys and two girls on the right-hand side of the picture is expressing encouragement and admiration. A group of two boys and two girls on the left-hand side of the picture is expressing fear (designed to pull for interpersonal relations, achievement motivation, and self-concept).

Card 17 B*: A boy is studying and daydreaming about receiving an *A* and an *F* from his teacher (designed to pull for anxiety/depression, achievement motivation, and self-concept).

Card 17 G*: A girl is studying and daydreaming about receiving an *A* and an *F* from her teacher (designed to pull for anxiety/depression, achievement motivation, and self-concept).

Card 18 B: A boy is studying and daydreaming about becoming an actor, a doctor, and a vagrant (designed to pull for achievement motivation and self-concept).

Card 18 G: A girl is studying and daydreaming about becoming an actress, a doctor, and a vagrant (designed to pull for achievement motivation and self-concept).

Exhibit continues

Exhibit 15.1.   (*Continued*)

Card 19 B: A boy in a window is imagining himself being saved from a burning building by a fireman and Superman (designed to pull for anxiety/depression and reality testing).

Card 19 G: A girl in a window is imagining herself being saved from a burning building by a fireman and Superman (designed to pull for anxiety/depression and reality testing).

Card 20: A youngster is in bed dreaming of a scene showing a horse on a hill, a river, and a path leading to a castle (designed to pull for anxiety/depression).

Card 21*: A youngster is in bed dreaming of a monster eating something and a monster making threats (designed to pull for aggression, anxiety/depression, and reality testing).

Card 22 B*: A boy is standing in front of a bathroom mirror imagining his face reflected in the mirror with attributes of both sexes (designed to pull for anxiety/depression, sexual identity, and reality testing).

Card 22 G*: A girl is standing in front of a bathroom mirror imagining her face reflected in the mirror with attributes of both sexes (designed to pull for anxiety/depression, sexual identity, and reality testing).

Card 23 B: A boy is rejected by his parents and imagines himself running away from home with luggage and standing on a bridge looking at the sea below (designed to pull for interpersonal relations and anxiety/depression).

Card 23 G: A girl is rejected by her parents and imagines herself running away from home with luggage and standing on a bridge looking at the sea below (designed to pull for interpersonal relations and anxiety/depression).

Note. From *TEMAS (Tell-Me-A-Story) Manual* (pp. 3–5), by G. Costantino, R. Malgady, and L. A. Rogler, 1988, Los Angeles, CA: Western Psychological Services. Copyright 1988 by Western Psychological Services. Adapted with permission of the publisher, Western Psychological Services, 12031 Wilshire Blvd., Los Angeles, CA 90025. Not to be reprinted in whole or in part for any additional purpose without the expressed, written permission of the publisher. All rights reserved.

the stimulus. Relationships is scored *1* if it is recognized and blank if it is not recognized; inquiries are scored *1* if they are unanswered and blank if they are all answered. Omissions and transformations are scored in accordance with the number of omissions and transformations of main character, secondary character, event, and setting.

All affective functions (e.g., happy, sad, and angry) are scored *1* if they are present in the narrative and left blank if they are not mentioned. Personality functions are scored on a Likert-type 4-point rating scale, with *1* representing the most maladaptive resolution of the conflict and *4*, the most adaptive. A personality function is scored as N when the particular function it represents cannot be scored. In accordance with the Sullivanian construct of selective inattention, this n scoring, which in TEMAS is called "selective attention," has been found to discriminate between normal and clinical African American, Hispanic, and White children. Results of this study show that a group of children with attention deficit hyperactivity disorder (ADHD) were significantly more likely than normal children to

Exhibit 15.2. The Tell-Me-A-Story Test Measures

Cognitive Functions
There are 18 cognitive functions that can be scored for each TEMAS protocol: reaction time (RT), total time (TT), fluency (FL), total omissions (OM), main character omissions (MCO), secondary character omissions (SCO), event omissions (EO), setting omissions (SO), total transformations (TRANS), main character transformations (MCT), secondary character transformations (SCT), event transformations (ET), setting transformations (ST), inquiries (INQ), relationships (REL), imagination (IMAG), sequencing (SEQ), and conflict (CON).

Personality Functions
Nine personality functions are assessed by TEMAS. Each stimulus card pulls for at least one of the following personality functions: interpersonal relations (IR), aggression (AGG), anxiety/depression (A/D), achievement motivation (AM), delay of gratification (DG), self-concept (SC), sexual identity (SEX), moral judgment (MJ), and reality testing (REAL).

Affective Functions
The TEMAS scoring system also evaluates seven affective functions: happy (HAP), sad (SAD), angry (ANG), fearful (FEAR), neutral (NEUT), ambivalent (AMB), and inappropriate affect (IA).

Note. From *TEMAS (Tell-Me-A-Story) Manual* (p. 5), by G. Costantino, R. Malgady, and L. A. Rogler, 1988, Los Angeles, CA: Western Psychological Services. Copyright 1988 by Western Psychological Services. Adapted with permission of the publisher, Western Psychological Services, 12031 Wilshire Blvd., Los Angeles, CA 90025. Not to be reprinted in whole or in part for any additional purpose without the expressed, written permission of the publisher. All rights reserved.

omit information in the TEMAS stimuli about characters, events and settings, and psychological conflicts. Differences between the groups were large and persistent in the presence of structured inquiries by the TEMAS examiners. Results of this study suggest the potential utility of TEMAS n scoring for the assessment of ADHD, thus facilitating *Diagnostic and Statistical Manual of Mental Disorders* (American Psychiatric Association, 1994) diagnosis. In addition, TEMAS n scoring, together with other clinical scores, have been found to significantly discriminate between normal and clinical groups of African American, Hispanic, and White children with 86% (for White) and 89% (for African American and Hispanic) classification accuracy (Cardalda, 1995; Costantino, Malgady, Colon-Malgady, & Bailey, 1992; Costantino, Malgady, Rogler, & Tsui, 1988).

A score of *1* for any personality function indicates a highly maladaptive resolution for a particular card. For example, references of murder, rape, and assault are scored *1* for interpersonal relations, aggression, and moral judgment. A suicidal theme earns a *1* under the anxiety/depression function. The decision to drop out of school or steal rather than work results in a *1* for achievement motivation and delay of gratification. The anticipation of complete failure and concomitant refusal to attempt a given task results in a *1* for self-concept of competence. A character who changes sexes or rejects his or her gender earns a *1* in sexual identity. The score of *1* in moral judgment reflects a severe lack of regard for the consequences of antisocial behavior.

Severely impaired reality testing is scored only for the most bizarre and impossible resolutions (e.g., inanimate objects come alive and kill, a child causes a harmful event to occur by a strange power of the mind). A score of 2 for any personality function reflects a moderately maladaptive resolution. Examples of such resolutions are a child cheats and gets away with it, a conflict is resolved by fighting, money is squandered rather than saved, homework is avoided in favor of play, a child runs away from home and never returns, and the monster in a dream might also be in the back-yard. A score of 3 represents a partially adaptive resolution. Examples of such resolutions are a child who cheats is caught and punished, fighting ceases in favor of compromise, money is saved for a time and then spent, homework is grudgingly completed, and a runaway child returns home.

A score of 4 represents a highly adaptive resolution. The child must perceive the intended conflict and solve the problem in a mature, age-appropriate manner. A score of 4 implies a striving for the greater good, a sense of responsibility, and an intrinsic motivation. Examples of such res-olutions are a child rejects the notion of cheating as contrary to learning, conflicts are discussed and a compromise is reached, money is saved for the future, homework is completed because good grades are valued, a child decides to talk to his or her parents rather than run away, and dreams are never real.

Standardization

The TEMAS was standardized on a sample of 642 children (281 boys and 361 girls) from the public schools in the New York City area. These chil-dren ranged in age from 5 to 13 years, with a mean age of 8.9 years (SD = 1.9). The total sample represented four ethnic–racial groups: Whites, Blacks, Puerto Ricans, and other Hispanics. Data on the socioeconomic status of the standardization sample indicate that these children were from predominantly lower- and middle-income families (Costantino, Mal-gady, & Rogler, 1988).

The TEMAS was administered to each child, with 23 cards presented in random order by an examiner of the same ethnic–racial background as the child. All children were tested individually by graduate psychology students in sessions conducted in a public school.

The nature of the distribution of some TEMAS functions made it im-practical to convert them to standard scores because scores other than zero were rare in the standardization sample. These functions are designated "qualitative indicators." The TEMAS functions, which had relatively nor-mal distributions, are designated "quantitative scales" (Costantino, Mal-gady, & Rogler, 1988).

Stratification of the Standardization Sample

In the same standardization sample, significant correlations of low mag-nitude were found between age and many of the TEMAS functions. Correlations ranged from .01 to .25, with a median value of .10. Although these correlations are small, it is believed that they reflect real developmental trends in children's cognitive, affective, and personality functioning. Thus, to accommodate the effects of these trends while still retaining respectable sample sizes, psychologists collapsed age into three year-range groups: 5- to 7-year-olds, 8- to 10-year-olds, and 11- to 13-year-olds.

For each of the 17 quantitative scales, three-way analyses of variance were computed by age, ethnic–racial background, and sex of the standardization sample. The three-way interaction terms were not significant for any of the quantitative functions. The two-way interactions between sex and age were also nonsignificant for these scales. The two-way interaction of sex and ethnic–racial background was significant for only one of the 17 quantitative scales, namely, sexual identity. However, given the number of variables tested, this result could be attributed to chance. There were no significant main effects of sex for any of these functions. This result is consistent with the results by other researchers who investigated the effects of gender on TEMAS functions (Cardalda, 1995; Elliot, 1998).

Means and standard deviations for the short form were derived by extracting the scores of the 9 cards from the 23-card protocols of the standardization sample. The correlations between the 23-card long form of the TEMAS and the 9-card short form for each function were computed separately for the total sample and for each ethnic–racial group. The correlation between the long form and the short form was uniformly high across samples. The median correlation between forms was .81 for the total sample, .82 for Whites, .80 for Blacks, .80 for Puerto Ricans, and .81 for other Hispanics.

Derivation of Standard Scores

To enable users to directly compare scores within a single protocol and to facilitate comparisons with the performance of the standardization sample, psychologists converted raw scores of quantitative scales to normalized T scores ($M = 50$, $SD = 10$). To minimize irregularities in the raw score distribution, psychologists also used an analytic smoothing technique (Cureton & Tukey, 1951). Because it was inappropriate to transform raw scores of the qualitative indicators to standard scores, critical levels based on the raw score distributions were provided, based on expert clinical opinion.

Reliability

In this context, *internal consistency* refers to the degree to which individual TEMAS cards are interrelated in measuring particular functions. Internal consistency reliabilities of the TEMAS long form functions were derived using a sample of 73 Hispanic and 42 Black children. The internal consistency reliability coefficients for the Hispanic sample ranged from .41 for ambivalent, an affective function, to .98 for fluency, a cognitive function, with a median value of .73. For the Black sample, coefficients ranged from .31 for setting transformations to .97 for fluency, with a median of .62.

Test–retest stability of the TEMAS functions was computed for the short form by correlating the results of two administrations, separated by an 18-week interval. The sample used in this study consisted of 51 students chosen at random from 210 Puerto Rican students screened for behavior problems. Results indicate that TEMAS functions exhibited low-to-moderate stability (r values ranging from .08 to .53) over an 18-week period. The eight TEMAS functions with significant test–retest correlations were fluency, event transformations, conflict, relationships, happy, neutral, anxiety/depression, and sexual identity. Three explanations for the generally low level of test–retest reliability were proposed. First, test–retest correlations may be lower bound estimates of reliability in this case because different raters were used at pre- and posttesting (Costantino, Malgady, & Rogler, 1988). Therefore, they include error variance due to interrater reliability. Second, the indicators of this instrument have limited range, and hence, the correlation may be attenuated. Third, the test–retest time interval was longer than usual, and children's developmental changes may have reduced the correlation.

Interrater Reliability

The protocols of 27 Hispanic and 26 Black children were drawn at random from the sample of 73 Hispanics and 42 Blacks described above in the section on internal consistency of the long form. Each protocol was scored independently by two raters. These scores were then correlated to estimate the degree to which the two raters agreed in their scoring of a particular picture for a given TEMAS personality function.

Interrater reliabilities in scoring total omissions (ranging from 0.33 to 1.00) and transformations (ranging from 0.32 to 1.00) were generally moderate-to-high for both the Hispanic and the Black protocols. Little difference was evident as a function of ethnic–racial group. For the affective functions, the pattern of correlation between raters was generally high (ranging from 0.70 to 1.00), with no substantive differences between the Hispanic and Black samples. With respect to the personality functions, correlations were low-to-moderate (ranging from .32 to .60) for reality testing and sexual identity in the Hispanic sample and overall substantially higher for the remaining functions (ranging from 0.30 to 1.00). Contrary to the pattern of internal consistency reliability estimates, the interrater reliabilities obtained for Hispanics were generally higher than for the Black sample.

Interrater reliability was also estimated in a more recent study of the nonminority version of the TEMAS short form (Costantino, Malgady, Casullo, & Castillo, 1991). Two experienced clinical psychologists (one with extensive training in scoring TEMAS and the other a newly trained scorer) independently rated 20 protocols. The results of this study indicate a higher interrater agreement in scoring protocols for personality functions, ranging from 75% to 95%. The mean level of interrater agreement was 81%, and in no cases were the two independent ratings different by more than 1 rating-scale point.

It is important to clarify that whereas the interrater agreement for personality functions in the first interrater reliability study ranged from 31% to 100%, in the more recent study the interrater agreement ranged from 75% to 95%. The explanation for this discrepancy may be that during the first study, which was conducted in 1983, the TEMAS scoring system was still undergoing changes, whereas in the second study, which was conducted in 1987, the scoring system and the instructions were completely formulated.

Content Validity

TEMAS pictures were designed to "pull" for specific personality functions based on the nature of the psychological conflict represented in each picture. As described above in the scoring section, all TEMAS pictures are scored for at least two personality functions. A study was conducted to assess the concordance among a sample of practicing school ($n = 8$) and clinical ($n = 6$) psychologists regarding the pulls of each TEMAS picture for specific personality functions. With respect to ethnicity, 7 clinicians were White, 1 was Black, and 6 were Hispanic. The clinical orientations of the psychologists in this sample included eclectic, psychoanalytic, cognitive, and ego psychology (Costantino, Malgady, & Rogler, 1988).

The psychologists were presented the TEMAS pictures in random order and were asked individually to indicate which, if any, of the nine personality functions were pulled by each picture. The percentage of agreement among the 14 clinicians revealed high agreement (71–100%) across the pictures, thus confirming the pulls scored for specific personality functions.

Relationship to Other Measures

A group of 210 Puerto Rican children screened for behavior problems were administered a number of measures along with the TEMAS, and their adaptive behavior in experimental role-playing situations was observed and rated by psychological examiners. The measures administered included the Sentence Completion Test of ego development (SCT; Loevinger & Wessler, 1970) or its Spanish version (Brenes-Jette, 1987); the Trait Anxiety Scale of the State–Trait Anxiety Inventory for Children (STAIC; Spielberger, Edwards, Lushene, Montuori, & Platzek, 1973) or its Spanish version, Inventario de Ansiedad Rasgo–Estado Para Niños (Villamil, 1973); and the Teacher Behavior Rating Scale (TBR; Costantino, 1978), and the parallel Mother Behavior Rating Scale (MBR; Costantino, 1978) in both English and Spanish. Finally, the children participated in four experimental role-playing situations, designed to elicit adaptive behavior.

Results of the regression analyses indicate that TEMAS profiles significantly predicted ego development (SCT), $R = .39$, $p < .05$; teachers' behavior ratings (TBR), $R = .49$, $p < .05$; delay of gratification (DG), $R = .32$, $p < .05$; self-concept of competence (SCC), $R = .50$, $p < .05$; disruptive behavior (DIS), $R = .51$, $p < .05$; and aggressive behavior (AGG), $R = .32$, $p < .05$. However, the multiple correlation for predicting trait anxiety was not significant. TEMAS functions accounted for between 10% (for DG and AGG) and 26% (for DIS) of the variability in scores on the criterion measures.

Predictive validity was established using hierarchical multiple regression analysis to assess the utility of TEMAS profiles for predicting posttherapy scores ($N = 123$) on the criterion measures, independent of pretherapy scores. In the first step of the hierarchy, the pretherapy score on a given criterion measure was entered into the regression equation, followed in the second step by a complete TEMAS pretherapy profile. Results of these analyses show that pretherapy TEMAS profiles significantly predicted all therapeutic outcomes, ranging from 6% to 22% increments in variance explained, except for observation of self-concept of competence. Several other studies have been conducted on TEMAS to assess its multicultural validity and clinical utility and show positive results (Bernal, 1991; Costantino, 1978; Costantino, Colon-Malgady, Malgady, & Perez, 1991; Costantino & Malgady, 1983; Costantino, Malgady, et al., 1991; Costantino et al., 1992; Costantino et al., 1981; Costantino, Malgady, Rogler, & Tsui, 1988; Elliot, 1998; Malgady, Costantino, & Rogler, 1984). The extent of this research points to a firm psychometric foundation for the TEMAS.

Conclusion

The TEMAS was developed as a multicultural test to "resuscitate the Thematic Apperception Test (TAT), . . . for children and adolescents, by providing a consensual scoring system" (Dana, 1996, p. 480). Culturally specific pictures for Hispanic and African Americans (minority version) and European Americans (nonminority version) and more recently pictures for Asian Americans depict culturally oriented and familiar interpersonal and intrapersonal situations and emic cultural symbols in an urban setting. The antithetical nature of the situation portrayed in the pictures pulls negative feelings from the test taker to be projected into a narrative content and manifested as an adaptive and maladaptive resolution of the underlying genotype conflict (Atkinson, 1981). These situations pull themes expressing various degrees of psychopathology (Costantino, Malgady, & Rogler, 1988). Welcomed as a "landmark event for multicultural assessment because it provides a picture story test that has psychometric credibility" (Dana, 1996, p. 480), the TEMAS has also been positively compared with the Rorschach comprehensive system as the only "projective methods that have established reliability and validity for multicultural assessment" (Ritzler, 1996, p. 120) and has contributed to nonbiased assessment of culturally and linguistically diverse children and adolescents in the United States, Central America, and South America (Barona & Hernandez, 1960; Bernal, 1991; Cardalda, 1995; Costantino, Malgady, Casullo, & Castillo, 1991; Walton, Nuttal, & Vaszquez-Nuttal, 1991). The TEMAS has greatly contributed to the revival of the TAT technique in cross-cultural and multicultural assessment; thus, the TEMAS embodies the appellative as the multicultural offspring of the TAT.

References

American Psychiatric Association. (1994). *Diagnostic and statistical manual of mental disorders* (4th ed.). Washington, DC: Author.

American Psychological Association. (1993). Guidelines for providers of psychological services to ethnic, linguistic, and culturally diverse populations. *American Psychologist, 4,* 45–48.

Ames, L. B., & August, J. (1966). Rorschach responses of Negro and White 5- to 10-year-olds. *Journal of Genetic Psychology, 10,* 297–309.

Anderson, H., & Anderson, G. (1955). *An introduction to projective techniques.* New York: Prentice Hall.

Anderson, M. P. (1981). Assessment of imaginal processes: Approaches and issues. In T. Merluzzi, C. Glass, & M. Genest (Eds.), *Cognitive assessment* (pp. 120–128). New York: Guilford Press.

Atkinson, H. W. (1981). Studying personality in the context of advanced motivational psychology. *American Psychologist, 36,* 117–128.

Auld, F. (1954). Contribution of behavior theory to projective testing. *Journal of Projective Techniques, 18,* 129–142.

Bailey, B. E., & Green, J., III. (1977). Black Thematic Apperception Test stimulus material. *Journal of Personality Assessment, 4,* 25–30.

Bandura, A. (1977). *Social learning theory.* Englewood Cliffs, NJ: Prentice Hall.

Bandura, A., & Walters, R. H. (1967). *Social learning and personality development.* New York: Holt, Rinehart, & Winston.

Barona, A., & Hernandez, A. E. (1990). Use of projective techniques in the assessment of Hispanic children. In A. Barona & E. E. Garcia (Eds.), *Children at risk: Poverty minority status and other issues in educational equity* (pp. 297–304). Washington, DC: National Association of School Psychologists.

Bellak, L. (1954). A study in limitations and "failures": Toward an ego psychology of projective techniques. *Journal of Projective Techniques, 10,* 279–293.

Bellak, L. (1989). *The TAT, CAT and SAT in clinical use* (5th ed.). New York: Grune & Stratton.

Bernal, I. (1991). *The relationship between level of acculturation, the Robert's Apperception Test for Children, and the TEMAS (Tell-Me-A-Story Test).* Doctoral dissertation, California School of Professional Psychology, Los Angeles.

Booth, L. J. (1966). A normative comparison of the responses of Latin American and Anglo American children to the Children's Apperception Test. In M. R. Haworth (Ed.), *The CAT: Facts about fantasy* (pp. 115–138). New York: Grune & Stratton.

Brenes-Jette, C. (1987). *Mother's contribution to an early intervention program for Hispanic children.* Unpublished dissertation, New York University, New York.

Cardalda, E. (1995). *Socio-cultural correlates to school achievement using the TEMAS (Tell-Me-A-Story) culturally sensitive test with sixth, seventh, and eighth graders.* Doctoral dissertation, New School for Social Research, New York.

Costantino, G. (1978, November). *TEMAS: A new thematic apperception test to measure ego functions and development in urban Black and Hispanic children.* Paper presented at the Second Annual Conference on Fantasy and the Imaging Process, Chicago.

Costantino, G., Colon-Malgady, G., Malgady, R. G., & Perez, A. (1991). Assessment of attention deficit disorder using a thematic apperception technique. *Journal of Personality Assessment, 57,* 87–95.

Costantino, G., & Malgady, R. G. (1983). Verbal fluency of Hispanic, Black and White children on TAT and TEMAS, a new thematic apperception test. *Hispanic Journal of Behavioral Sciences, 5,* 199–206.

Costantino, G., & Malgady, R. (1995). Development of TEMAS, a multicultural thematic apperception test: Psychometric properties and clinical utility. In G. R. Sodowsky & J. C. Impara (Eds.), *Multicultural assessment in counseling and clinical psychology* (pp. 85–136). Lincoln: University of Nebraska, Buros Institute of Mental Measurements.

Costantino, G., Malgady, R., Casullo, M. M., & Castillo, A. (1991). Cross-cultural standardization of TEMAS in three Hispanic subcultures. *Hispanic Journal of Behavioral Sciences, 13,* 48–62.

Costantino, G., Malgady, R. G., Colon-Malgady, G., & Bailey, J. (1992). Clinical utility of the TEMAS with non-minority children. *Journal of Personality Assessment, 59,* 433–438.

Costantino, G., Malgady, R., & Rogler, L. H. (1988). *TEMAS (Tell-Me-A-Story) manual.* Los Angeles, CA: Western Psychological Services.

Costantino, G., Malgady, R. G., Rogler, L. H., & Tsui, E. (1988). Discriminant analysis of clinical outpatients and public school children by TEMAS: A thematic apperception test for Hispanics and Blacks. *Journal of Personality Assessment, 52,* 670–678.

Costantino, G., Malgady, R. G., & Vazquez, C. (1981). A comparison of the Murray TAT and a new thematic apperception test for urban Hispanic children. *Hispanic Journal of Behavioral Sciences, 3,* 291–300.

Cureton, E. E., & Tukey, J. W. (1951). Smoothing frequency distribution, equating tests, and preparing norms. *American Psychologist, 6,* 404–410.

Dana, R. H. (1986). Personality assessment and native Americans. *Journal of Personality Assessment, 50,* 480–500.

Dana, R. H. (1993). *Multicultural assessment perspectives for professional psychology.* Boston: Allyn & Bacon.

Dana, R. H. (1996). Culturally competent assessment practice in the United States. *Journal of Personality Assessment, 66,* 472–487.

Durret, M. E., & Kim, C. C. (1973). A comparative study of behavioral maturity in Mexican American and Anglo preschool children. *Journal of Genetic Psychology, 123,* 55–62.

Elliot, T. L. (1998). *Differential validation of the TEMAS (Tell-Me-A-Story) with Rorschach as criterion: A comparison of projective method.* Unpublished doctoral dissertation, Long Island University, New York.

Exner, J. E., & Weiner, I. B. (1982). *The Rorschach: A comprehensive system. Vol. 3: Assessment of children and adolescents.* New York: Wiley.

Forgus, R., & Shulman, B. (1979). *Personality: A cognitive view.* Englewood Cliffs, NJ: Prentice Hall.

Gallager, J. J. (1979). Research centers and social policy. *American Psychologist, 34,* 997–1000.

Holt, R. R. (1960a). Cognitive controls and primary processes. *Journal of Psychological Researches, 4,* 105–112.

Holt, R. R. (1960b). Recent developments in psychoanalytic ego psychology and their implications for diagnostic testing. *Journal of Projective Techniques, 24,* 251–266.

Kagan, J. (1956). The measurement of overt aggression from fantasy. *Journal of Abnormal Social Psychology, 52,* 390–393.

Loevinger, J., & Wessler, R. (1970). *Measuring ego development. 1. Construction and use of a sentence completion test.* San Francisco: Jossey-Bass.

Malgady, R. G. (1996). The question of cultural bias in assessment and diagnosis of ethnic minority clients: Let's reject the null hypothesis. *Professional Psychology: Research and Practice, 27,* 101–105.

Malgady, R. G., Costantino, G., & Rogler, L. H. (1984). Development of a thematic apperception test (TEMAS) for urban Hispanic children. *Journal of Consulting and Clinical Psychology, 52,* 986–996.

Murray, H. A. (1943). *The Thematic Apperception Test: Manual.* Cambridge, MA: Harvard University Press.

Murray, H. A. (1951). Uses of the Thematic Apperception Test. *American Journal of Psychiatry, 107,* 577–581.

Murstein, B. I. (1963). *Theory and research in projective techniques.* New York: Wiley.

Padilla, A. M. (1979). Critical factors in the testing of Hispanic Americans: A review and some suggestions for the future. In R. Tyler & S. White (Eds.), *Testing, teaching and learning: Report of a conference on testing* (pp. 219–243). Washington, DC: National Institute of Education.

Paivio, A. (1971). *Imagery and verbal processes.* New York: Holt, Rinehart, & Winston.

Piaget, J., & Inhelder, B. (1971). *Mental imagery in the child.* New York: Basic Books.

Reuman, D. A., Alvin, D. F., & Veroff, J. (1983, August). *Measurement models for thematic apperceptive measure of achievement motive.* Paper presented at the 91st Annual Convention of the American Psychological Association, Anaheim, CA.

Ritzler, B. (1996). Multicultural projective assessment: Rorschach, TEMAS, and the early memories procedures. In L. A. Suzuki, P. J. Meller, & J. J. Ponterotto (Eds.), *Handbook for multicultural assessment* (pp. 114–135). San Francisco: Jossey-Bass.

Singer, J. L., & Pope, K. (Eds.). (1978). *The power of human imagination: New methods in psychotherapy.* New York: Plenum Press.

Sobel, J. J. (1981). Projective methods of cognitive analysis. In T. Merluzzi, G. Glass, & M. Genest (Eds.), *Cognitive assessment* (pp. 127–148). New York: Garfield Press.

Spielberger, C. D., Edwards, C. D., Lushene, R. E., Montuori, J., & Platzek, D. (1973). *Preliminary test manual for the State–Trait Anxiety Inventory for Children.* Palo Alto, CA: Consulting Psychologists Press.

Thompson, C. E. (1949). The Thompson modification of the Thematic Apperception Test. *Journal of Projective Techniques, 17,* 469–478.

Villamil, B. (1973). *Desarrollo del inventario de ansiesad estado y rasgo para ninos* [Development of the State–Trait Anxiety Inventory for Children]. Unpublished master's thesis, University of Puerto Rico, San Juan.

Walton, J., Nuttall, R. R., & Vazquez-Nuttall, E. (1997). The impact of war on the mental health of children: A Salvadoran study. *Child Abuse & Neglect, 21,* 737–749.

16

The Thematic Apperception Test and the Multivoiced Nature of the Self

Hubert J. M. Hermans

In this chapter, I describe my proposal for integrating Thematic Apperception Test (TAT) interpretation with my narrative therapy approach. The commonality of storytelling in response to the TAT cards and of storytelling in the course of narrative therapy is discussed. Emphasis is placed on the "polyphonic" perspective from which the TAT can be interpreted to better understand the multivoiced nature of the individual self. I show how this form of interpretation is in concert with Murray's views of the TAT and personality.

Self-Confrontation Method

I was interested in understanding each individual's unique construction of personal meaning or "human valuation." Phenomenological research led me to devise a new instrument, the *self-confrontation method,* which invites people to tell stories about their lives and to focus on those parts in their past, present, or future that had a particular personal meaning for them. Take, for example, three statements such as "Last year I lost my wife in an accident," "I am now involved in a project which absorbs all my attention," and "In the future, I hope to find a mutually stimulating relationship with a partner." I conceived these statements as valuations representing important personal meaning units. As part of the self-confrontation method, I present a list of feelings to the person with the instruction to rate the affective characteristics of each of the valuations. The main distinction is between self-enhancing feelings (e.g., self-esteem, strength, and self-confidence) and feelings referring to contact and union (e.g., tenderness, intimacy, and love). This enables me to assess two basic motives (striving for self-enhancement and longing for contact and union) for each valuation separately. In experimenting with this device, I made one of my most dramatic discoveries: investigating people's self-narratives also changes these narratives. Inviting people to formulate valuations and investigating the underlying motivation not only worked as an assessment of the valuation system but also as a means to stimulate it toward therapeutic change (Hermans & Hermans-Jansen, 1995).

My goal here is to outline a proposal for future use of the TAT. This proposal is based on a deep commonality between the TAT and the self-confrontation method in a narrative psychotherapy approach. The quintessence of my proposal is to assume that the storyteller (the patient) projects his or her needs not to one single hero in the story but to a multiplicity of heroes.

To better understand this proposal, I now return to some of Murray's (1943) original guidelines for interpreting the stories told in response to TAT pictures. First, the psychologist identifies the hero in the story, usually the person who most resembles the storyteller. Second, the psychologist considers the hero's motives, trends, and feelings; careful attention has to be paid to the story's content as disclosing the client's particular needs. Third, the psychologist analyzes the forces (known as *presses*) in the hero's environment that provide or block opportunities for need expression. Along these lines, the psychologist receives an impression of the dynamic interplay between needs and presses in the client's story.

I propose that the three guidelines are followed not only for the main hero of a story but also for a secondary hero or heroes. The secondary hero is portrayed by the client as an antagonist. The assumption is that the antagonist also belongs to the client's self as a dynamic, multivoiced entity (Hermans, 1996a, 1996b; also see Rosenzweig, chap. 4, this volume, regarding his composite portrait method of TAT analysis, in which he seemed to have anticipated my approach). The protagonist and the antagonist represent separate voices, which are able to tell specific stories about themselves in relation to the perceived environment. Each voice tells a particular story with specific needs and presses.

It is therefore recommended that after the storyteller completes telling stories for the TAT cards, he or she should go back over the cards and where there is one or more antagonist or secondary hero–heroine, he or she should make up a story from that person's point of view. In doing so, storytellers are instructed just as they were instructed at the beginning— to tell a story about what happened before the scene in the picture, what is going on at the present time, what the people are thinking and feeling, and what the outcome will be. These stories are then compared and analyzed in conjunction with the first story in which there was a single hero or heroine with whom the storyteller identified. Patient and therapist collaborate in TAT interpretation (an approach also advocated by Bellak, see chap. 11, this volume). I derived this approach on the basis of my clinical work as well as from Bakhtin's (1929/1973) concept of the *polyphonic novel*.

The Polyphonic Novel:
Differences Between Logical and Dialogical Relationships

The Russian literary scholar Mikhail Bakhtin (1929/1973) asserted that Dostoyevsky introduced a new artistic form, the polyphonic novel. The principal feature of the polyphonic novel is that it is composed of a number of independent and mutually opposing viewpoints embodied by characters involved in dialogical relationships. The characters are not to be seen as "obedient slaves" in the service of Dostoyevsky's artistic intentions but are capable of standing beside their creator (author), disagreeing with the author, and even rebelling against him. The polyphonic novel rejects the idea of an omniscient author who is "above" his characters and understands them from a highly centralized viewpoint. Instead, each character is "ideologically authoritative and independent" (Bakhtin, 1929/1973, p. 3). Each character is perceived as the author of his or her own legitimate ideological position.

Bakhtin maintained that in Dostoyevsky's novels there is not one single author but several authors or thinkers. Each character, such as Myshkin, Stavogin, Raskolnikov, Ivan Karamazov, and the Grand Inquisitor, has his own voice and tells his own story. When different characters meet one another, they respond to one another in what Bakhtin calls a *dialogical fashion*: As in a polyphonic composition, several voices or instruments have different spatial positions and accompany and oppose each other in a dialogical relation. In Bakhtin's (1929/1973) dialogical view,

> consciousness is never self-sufficient; it always finds itself in an intense relationship with another consciousness. The hero's every experience and his every thought is internally dialogical, polemically colored and filled with opposing forces . . . open to inspiration from outside itself. (p. 26)

The voices of Dostoyevsky's heroes are continuously resisting any final (i.e., closed, logical) conclusion: "Every thought of Dostoyevsky's heroes . . . feels itself to be a speech in an uncompleted dialog" (p. 27). Unfinalizability and openness, as intrinsic features of dialogue, are necessary conditions for the understanding of individual lives.

Bakhtin (1929/1973) observed that Dostoyevsky's world is "profoundly personalized" and that each character is a "concrete consciousness, embodied in the living voice of an integral person" (p. 7). Bakhtin therefore emphasized that a particular utterance should never be isolated from the consciousness of a particular character. Moreover, one particular character is always implicitly or explicitly responding to another character; therefore, "a dialogical reaction personifies every utterance to which it reacts" (p. 152).

According to Bakhtin (1929/1973), Dostoyevsky's novels present a spatial construction of reality in which readers simultaneously hear a plurality of voices representing a plurality of worlds that are neither identical nor unified but rather heterogeneous and even opposed. Within this spatial world of sounds, Dostoyevsky portrayed characters conversing with the devil (Ivan and the Devil), their alter egos (Ivan and Smerdyakov), and even caricatures of themselves (Raskolnikov and Svidrigailov).

As in a musical polyphonic composition, a particular idea or theme (e.g., aggression, love, jealousy, tenderness) does not have a fixed, self-contained, unchangeable meaning; it is not bound to a fixed, centralized perspective. Instead, by leading the theme through the various voices, its many facets and potentials can be brought to expression.

The Polyphonic Novel as a Metaphor for the Thematic Apperception Test

A TAT card can be regarded as a pictorial version of a polyphonic novel. Each of the actors in an individual's TAT stories has his or her own story and may tell a specific story about his or her own past, present, or future, resulting in highly personal themes that constitute the unique self of the individual (see also Cramer, 1996). Different characters play their part in the story a person tells about himself or herself with these characters expressing psychological motives that make up the multiplicity of the self's voices (Hermans & Kempen, 1993).

Consider Card 8 BM (the operation scene). In a story of this picture, needs and presses are analyzed only from the perspective of the hero, usually the young man in the foreground who may be seen as considering a career in medicine. In my approach, when the storyteller selects the antagonist, such as the surgeon in this picture, the storyteller is then asked to make up a story for the picture from the point of view of the antagonist–surgeon. In the situation I am describing, for example, the storyteller who identified with the young man sees the surgeon as the young man's father who wants him to pursue a career that he does not want to follow. From the position of the father, however, the client may tell about the father's hope that his son will also pursue a career as a surgeon. Because the two positions are evoked by the same picture, the client may focus on the tension between the two stories, which may reveal a conflict within himself or herself. Awareness of this conflict is stimulated by shifting between both perspectives and by considering them simultaneously. In this manner, the storyteller behaves in a multivoiced manner, extending his or her apperception of the situation beyond the perception of just one position—all of which provides good material for use in psychotherapy.

By viewing the alternation between positions, storytellers when in psychotherapy may be helped to confront the conflicts, negotiations, agreements, and disagreements that are so typical of the dialogical functioning of the self. Using the TAT in therapy to focus on the different perspectives may well lead to a broadening of viewpoints in the direction of a multiplicity of perspectives that receive coherence by the act of storytelling. Such a process of positioning and repositioning is an important starting point, or part, of any form of counseling or therapy that contributes to the extension and flexibility of the self, as does any self-confrontation approach.

My proposed procedure is well in agreement with some of Murray's ground-breaking views, including his belief that the TAT should be used therapeutically (see Gieser & Stein, chap. 1, this volume) and that TAT stories are related to literature (see Gieser & Morgan, chap. 5, this volume). One may even argue that Murray himself proposed a multivoiced view of the self, as the following passage suggests:

> I visualize . . . a whispering gallery in which voices echo from the distant past; a gulf stream of fantasies with floating memories of past events, currents of contending complexes, plots and counterplots, hopeful intimations and ideals. . . . A personality is a full Congress of orators and pressure groups of children, demagogues, communists, isolationists, war-mongers, mugwumps, grafters, logrollers, lobbyists, Caesars and Christs, Machiavellis and Judases, Tories and Promethean revolutionists. And a psychologist who does not know this in himself, whose mind is locked against the flux of images and feelings, should be encouraged to make friends, by being psychoanalyzed, with the various members of his household. (Murray, 1940, pp. 160–161)

References

Bakhtin, M. (1973). *Problems of Dostoyevsky's poetics* (2nd ed., R. W. Rotsel, Trans.). Ann Arbor, MI: Ardis. (Original work published 1929)

Cramer, P. (1996). *Storytelling, narrative, and the Thematic Apperception Test.* New York: Guilford Press.

Hermans, H. J. M. (1996a). Opposites in a dialogical self: Constructs as characters. *Journal of Constructivist Psychology, 9,* 1–26.

Hermans, H. J. M. (1996b). Voicing the self: From information processing to dialogical interchange. *Psychological Bulletin, 119,* 31–50.

Hermans, H. J. M., & Hermans-Jansen, E. (1995). *Self-narratives: The construction of meaning in psychotherapy.* New York: Guilford Press.

Hermans, H. J. M., & Kempen, H. J. G. (1993). *The dialogical self: Meaning as movement.* San Diego, CA: Academic Press.

Murray, H. A. (1940). What should psychologists do about psychoanalysis? *Journal of Abnormal and Social Psychology, 35,* 150–175.

Murray, H. A. (1943). *The Thematic Apperception Test: Manual.* Cambridge, MA: Harvard University Press.

Part VI

Conclusion

17

A View to the Future

Lon Gieser and Morris I. Stein

The Thematic Apperception Test (TAT) is the best compass for guiding psychologists in their explorations of personality. It differs significantly from other psychological assessment techniques: The TAT is ennobling by virtue of its focus on imagination, creativity, and stories (see chaps. 3, 5, and 6, this volume). People's lives are composed of stories as they continuously give meaning to their experiences and innerselves. They communicate with one another primarily by telling stories. Much of one's self-identity may be influenced by one's life story, or *personal narrative*, that one constructs for oneself as well as by the traditional stories of one's culture. The storytelling enterprise of the TAT therefore addresses the heart of our humanity. The TAT has been incorporated into "the narrative study of human lives" (McAdams, Diamond, de St. Aubin, & Mansfield, 1997, p. 679) in personality research. The TAT approach will undoubtedly be further advanced within this growing field of inquiry (see Cramer, 1996; Hermans, chap. 16; and McClelland, chap. 13, this volume).

Despite our admiration of the TAT, we do not believe it to be self-sufficient. The TAT can best contribute to psychological knowledge when its findings are integrated with multiple sources of data into a meaningful pattern. Data may be attained by Murray's "multiform method" or a standard test battery (see Anastasi, 1996; Groth-Marnat, 1997; Holt, chap. 8, this volume; and Teglasi, 1993). The TAT's use may be combined with biographical interviews and pertinent questionnaires and tests in accordance with the psychologist's needs for the case at hand, as is exemplified by Stein's (1981) manual–textbook (see chap. 10, this volume). The fields of neuropsychology, forensics, and cross-cultural study, in particular, continue to benefit from the unique data the TAT adds to other measures (see Bellak, chap. 11, this volume; Bellak & Abrams, 1997; Costantino & Malgady, chap. 15; and Dana, chap. 14, this volume). We concur with Murray (1943/1971) that *"the conclusions that are reached by an analysis of TAT stories must be regarded as good 'leads' or working hypotheses to be verified by other methods, rather than as proved facts"* (p. 17, emphasis in original; also see Karon, 1981, for an interpretive strategy that fosters hypothesis generation).

Reliance on projective techniques has decreased as strong belief in the psychoanalytic theory with which they have been traditionally allied has waned among many psychologists. The TAT, however, is amenable to diverse theoretical and practical orientations. One need not adhere to psychoanalysis or Murray's personology to use the TAT. One need only experience the TAT's transtheoretical capacity to elicit valuable information on psychological functioning beyond that obtained in direct interviews and structured tests and questionnaires (see Abrams, chap. 12, this volume). The current cognitive-neuropsychiatric zeitgeists need not leave the TAT in the dust. What other instrument can better help to further understand "emotional intelligence"?

Some psychologists consider the TAT to be a type of clinical interview (Obrzut & Cummings, 1983; Rossini & Moretti, 1997) rather than a test. Given the TAT's potential to facilitate emotional communication, we hope that its role as a psychotherapeutic tool gains greater recognition. Perhaps further integration of psychodynamic, cognitive, and narrative therapies will bring about more collaborative therapist–client interpretations. In psychotherapy with some clients without the necessity of scoring or report writing, the TAT may be used more freely in the service of the individual (see Bellak, chap. 11; Gieser & Stein, chap. 1; Hermans, chap. 16; and Rosenzweig, chap. 4, this volume).

Far too often, academic psychology has fallen prey to *methodolotry*—devoting more energy to the study of research instruments themselves than to substantive issues. There continues to be a disproportionate amount of research on the TAT itself—its validity, reliability, scoring, and other psychometrics—as compared with its role in understanding important psychological phenomena.

Empirical Evidence

Research on the TAT usually focuses on one or two personality variables at a time (e.g., needs, defenses, aggression). In statistical studies of group trends, these variables are studied across individuals, enabling psychologists to learn more about the variables. Individual persons are seldom studied across variables, as in *Explorations in Personality* (Murray, 1938). Psychologists are unnecessarily deprived of learning more about the complex interplay of personality variables within the psyches of warm-blooded individuals (see Anderson, chap. 3; and Gieser & Stein, chap. 1, this volume).

The most famous comprehensive study in the tradition of *Explorations in Personality* using both statistical and case study methods was reported in *The Authoritarian Personality* (Adorno, Frenkel-Brunswick, Levinson, & Sanford, 1950). It is common knowledge that authoritarianism is measured by the F Scale questionnaire (which also fell prey to methodolotry). Few realize that the F Scale is merely a convenient measure based on findings from interviews, projective tests, and other questionnaires. Nevitt Sanford, one of the F Scale's originators, once told one of us (Gieser) that given a choice between studying authoritarianism without the F Scale or the TAT, he would drop the F Scale in a minute.

The TAT is invaluable in linking the prejudicial individual to the authoritarian syndrome. A good example is the insight it provides regarding one's relationship to one's parents. The interviews and some questionnaire responses show that a distinguishable feature of highly prejudicial individuals was their tendency to glorify their parents (Adorno et al., 1950; Gieser, 1980; Sanford, 1973). But usually not long after statements of glorification, "a note of complaint or self-pity began to creep into the interview" (Sanford, 1973, p. 142).

By using the TAT, Adorno et al. (1950) were able to demonstrate that overt glorification of parents is functionally related to hostility toward them. The frequency and intensity of aggressive actions by the heroes in the TAT stories are, for the most part, indications of aggression, which is accepted by the individuals. Such aggression was pronounced in the TAT protocols of the less prejudicial individuals. The greater repressed conscious aggression against parents by highly prejudicial individuals was revealed by the frequency and intensity of aggression against parental figures on the part of nonheroic characters with whom the individual did not readily identify. There still is need for further validation of this finding because authoritarianism is no longer studied in this comprehensive manner using the TAT.

Another example of the TAT's value in personality study is the brilliant use of McClelland's (1975; also see McClelland, chap. 13; and Winter, chap. 9, this volume) adaptation of the TAT by Pollak and Gilligan (1982). Male and female college students wrote imaginative stories in response to McClelland's pictures. The observation of violence in men's stories about intimacy led to a comparative analysis of men's and women's fears pertaining to achievement and affiliation. This analysis revealed that the men projected more danger into situations of close, personal affiliation than into achievement situations. They associated danger with intimacy, expressing a fear of being caught in a smothering relationship or humiliated by rejection or deceit. In contrast, the women saw more danger in interpersonal achievement than in personal affiliation and connected danger with the isolation that they associated with constructive success. These contrasting perceptions of safety and danger in attachment and separation led to the identification of intimacy as the corollary to fear of success.

Despite methodological critics, Gilligan and Pollak (1988) later administered five of McClelland's TAT cards to male and female 1st-year medical students and interviewed the students to assess self-definition and moral judgment. Students were also questioned regarding stresses encountered in providing medical treatment and meeting the ideals of medicine and their aspirations. Both the TAT and interview responses were analyzed for themes of achievement, intimacy, and isolation. The TAT findings—images of success and failure and of intimacy and isolation—deepened an understanding of the interview material regarding these issues. As in Pollak and Gilligan's (1982) previous study, men tended to perceive relationships as potentially dangerous, whereas women tended to view relationships as safe. Women focused more frequently than did men on the dangers of isolation, whereas men tended to consider more saliently the risks of connection. Implications of these findings for helping medical students develop a psychological perspective that links achievement with attachment were offered by Gilligan and Pollak. McClelland's TAT was thus used empathically to further humanize the personal and professional selves of individuals.

Cramer (1998) presented an encouraging approach to learning about the TAT while developing clinical sensitivity[1]: "The areas of theory, clinical practice, research, and personal experience are used continually to illustrate and to inform each other" (p. 247). Interpretation of the relationship between TAT story themes and life history themes was taught by Morgan and Murray (1935) and the recent "more systematic" work of Demorest and Alexander (1992). Multiple perspectives from which to interpret TAT stories can be drawn from narrative theory (Bruner, 1986; Sarbin, 1986; Schafer, 1992; Spence, 1982). Classic case studies by White (1938), Keniston (1963), Murray (1955/1981), and Barron (1972) demonstrate the role of thematic analysis in depth assessment of individual personalities. Students are shown TAT coding approaches to assess personality motives (achievement, affiliation, power and intimacy; McAdams, 1988; McClelland, Atkinson, Clark, & Lowell, 1953; Shipley & Veroff, 1952; Smith, 1992; Stewart, 1982; Winter, 1973) as well as to assess gender identity (May, 1980), defense mechanisms (Cramer, 1991, 1995, 1996, 1997), and object relations (Westen, 1991).

Cramer's exercises and workshops using the TAT and McClelland's research series of cards (McClelland & Steele, 1972) focus on self-exploration, differential diagnosis, and general personality assessment, including how to discern the different levels of personality—traits (Level 1), motives or defenses (Level 2), and life themes or individual identity (Level 3; McAdams, 1995)—and the differences between self-attributed and implicit motives (McClelland, Koestner, & Weinberger, 1989). Relationships between personality variables and between projective and objective measures have been studied, especially with regard to predicting behavior.

Important longitudinal research using the TAT continues to be conducted at the Institute for Human Development at the University of California, Berkeley, and at the Henry A. Murray Research Center at Radcliffe College and the University of Michigan. Scientific study of personality traits and motives throughout the life span will most probably be enhanced by the use of the TAT for years to come (see Winter, John, Stewart, Kohen, & Duncan, 1998).

Conclusion

The TAT has proven to be eminently flexible and adaptable to a variety of clinical and research purposes (see chaps. 2, 4, 7, 10, 11, 12, 14, and 16, this volume). There is not only Murray's traditional TAT but also several

---

[1]We strongly recommend this chapter as well as Cramer's (1996) book, which covers well the domains of TAT interpretation, studies of clinical patients and of normal development, and research issues.

derivatives, with others most probably on the way (see chaps. 9, 10, and 13, this volume). *TAT* is now a generic term referring to a method for getting individuals to tell stories about pictures to learn about their personalities. (Similarly, the Rorschach, Behn–Rorschach, and Holtzman Inkblot Tests are all inkblot methods, each having its own rationale and scoring scheme.)

Therefore, in one form or another, the TAT is here to stay. It certainly will not become extinct so long as graduate students are required to write dissertations on such topics as test reliability and validity. The predictive validity of McClelland's TAT measure (vs. self-report questionnaires) has been impressive with regard to long-term behaviorial trends (see Cramer, 1996; McClelland, chap. 13; and Winter, chap. 9, this volume). Admirable efforts continue to be made toward bringing the TAT and its offspring increased psychometric respectability (see Abrams, chap. 12; Costantino & Malgady, chap. 15; and Dana, chap. 14, this volume). The field of clinical judgment research, which studies the relative accuracy of clinical inference versus statistical–actuarial methods in psychological assessment, has provided fertile ground for investigating the TAT's problematic validity, especially when interpretation is not based on quantified scoring systems and normative data (Garb, 1984, 1998a, 1998b; Klein, 1986; Lanyon & Goodstein, 1982; Ryan, 1985).

Nevertheless, we believe that the TAT's validity may best be determined by looking at how helpful it is to *well-trained psychologists in their particular areas of expertise*. Our concern is with how much individualized (i.e., nonformulaic) interpretations add to substantive knowledge about areas in which the interpretations are made. According to Teglasi (1993), the TAT lends itself

> to analysis through various approaches. The narrative process, content, and structure of the protocol can be looked at through different lenses, each revealing shades and nuances pertaining to a given facet of personality. As a result, no single scoring system can exhaust the rich and diverse possibilities for interpretation. (p. viii)

Different topic areas provide different perspectives from which to view TAT stories (see Abrams, chap. 12; Hermans, chap. 16; Rosenzweig, chap. 4; and Shneidman, chap. 7, this volume). Interpretation involves judgment based on a concurrent understanding of the phenomenon measured. With this sort of situational validity, the methodological line of inquiry becomes "How valid is the TAT under what circumstances?" (Shneidman, 1992). Ultimately, we arrive at Murray's (1943/1971) conclusion that "the future of the TAT hangs more on the possibility of perfecting the interpreter (psychology's forgotten instrument) more than it does on perfecting the material" (p. 8).

References

Adorno, T. W., Frenkel-Brunswick, E., Levinson, D. G., & Sanford, N. (1950). *The authoritarian personality*. New York: Harper & Row.

Anastasi, A. (1996). *Psychological testing* (7th ed.). New York: Macmillan.

Barron, F. (1972). *Artists in the making*. New York: Seminar Press.

Bellak, L., & Abrams, D. (1997). *The TAT, CAT, and SAT in clinical use* (6th ed.). Needham Heights, MA: Allyn & Bacon.

Bruner, J. (1986). *Actual minds, possible worlds*. Cambridge, MA: Harvard University Press.

Cramer, P. (1991). *The development of defense mechanisms*. New York: Springer-Verlag.

Cramer, P. (1995). Identity, narcissism and defense mechanisms in late adolescence. *Journal of Research in Personality, 29*, 341–361.

Cramer, P. (1996). *Storytelling, narrative and the Thematic Apperception Test*. New York: Guilford Press.

Cramer, P. (1997). Evidence for change in children's use of defense mechanisms. *Journal of Personality, 65*, 233–247.

Cramer, P. (1998). Approaching the Thematic Apperception Test (TAT). In L. Handler & M. J. Hilsenroth (Eds.), *Teaching and learning personality assessment* (pp. 247–265). Mahwah, NJ: Erlbaum.

Demorest, A. P., & Alexander, I. E. (1992). Affective scripts as organizers of personal experience. *Journal of Personality, 60*, 645–663.

Garb, H. N. (1984). The incremental validity of information used in personality assessment. *Clinical Psychology Review, 4*, 641–655.

Garb, H. N. (1998a). Recommendations for training in the use of the Thematic Apperception Test. *Professional Psychology: Research and Practice, 29*, 621–622.

Garb, H. N. (1998b). *Studying the clinician: Judgment research and psychological assessment*. Washington, DC: American Psychological Association.

Gieser, M. T. (1980). *"The authoritarian personality" revisited*. Berkeley, CA: The Wright Institute.

Gilligan, C., & Pollak, S. (1988). The vulnerable and invulnerable physician. In C. Gilligan, J. V. Ward, J. M. Taylor, & B. Badige (Eds.), *Mapping the moral domain: A contribution of women's thinking to psychological theory and education* (pp. 244–262). Cambridge, MA: Harvard University Press.

Groth-Marnat, G. (1997). *Handbook of psychological assessment* (3rd ed.). New York: Wiley.

Karon, B. P. (1981). The Thematic Apperception Test. In A. I. Rubin (Ed.), *Assessment with projective techniques: A concise introduction* (pp. 85–120). New York: Springer.

Keniston, K. (1963). Inburn: An American Ishmael. In R. White (Eds), *The study of lives* (pp. 40–70). New York: Atherton.

Klein, R. G. (1986). Questioning the usefulness of projective psychological tests for children. *Journal of Developmental and Behavioral Pediatrics, 7*, 378–382.

Lanyon, R. I., & Goodstein, L. D. (1982). *Personality assessment* (2nd ed.). New York: Wiley.

May, R. R. (1980). *Sex and fantasy: Patterns of male and female development*. New York: Norton.

McAdams, D. P. (1988). *Power, intimacy and the life story*. New York: Guilford Press.

McAdams, D. P. (1995). What do we know when we know a person? *Journal of Personality, 63*, 365–396.

McAdams, D. P., Diamond, A., de St. Aubin, E., & Mansfield, E. (1997). Stories of commitment: The psychosocial construction of generative lives. *Journal of Personality and Social Psychology, 72*, 678–694.

McClelland, D. C. (1975). *Power: The inner experience*. New York: Irving.

McClelland, D. C., Atkinson, J. W., Clark, R. A., & Lowell, E. L. (1953). *The achievement motive*. New York: Appleton-Century-Crofts.

McClelland, D. C., Koestner, R., & Weinberger, J. (1989). How do self-attributed and implicit motives differ? *Psychological Review, 96*, 690–702.

McClelland, D. C., & Steele, R. S. (1972). *Motivation workshops*. Morristown, NJ: General Learning Press.

Morgan, C. D., & Murray, H. (1935). A method for investigating fantasies: The Thematic Apperception Test. *Archives of Neurological Psychiatry, 3*, 115–143.

Murray, H. A. (Ed). (1938). *Explorations in personality: A clinical and experimental study of fifty college men*. New York: Oxford University Press.

Murray, H. A. (1971). *Thematic Apperception Test: Manual*. Cambridge, MA: Harvard University Press. (Original work published 1943)

Murray, H. A. (1981). American Icarus. In E. S. Shneidman (Ed.), *Endeavors in psychology: Selections from the personology of Henry A. Murray* (pp. 535–556). New York: Harper & Row. (Original work published 1955)

Obrzut, J. E., & Cummings, J. A. (1983). The projective approach to personality assessment: An analysis of thematic picture techniques. *School Psychology Review, 12,* 414–420.

Pollak, S., & Gilligan, C. (1982). Images of violence in Thematic Apperception Test stories. *Journal of Personality and Social Psychology, 42,* 159–167.

Rossini, E. D., & Moretti, R. J. (1997). Thematic Apperception Test (TAT) interpretation: Practice recommendations from a survey of clinical psychology doctoral programs accredited by the American Psychological Association. *Professional Psychology: Research and Practice, 28,* 393–398.

Ryan, R. M. (1985). Thematic Apperception Test. In D. J. Keyser & R. C. Sweetland (Eds.), *Test critiques* (Vol. 2, pp. 799–814). Kansas City, MO: Test Corporation of America.

Sanford, N. (1973). The authoritarian personality in contemporary perspective. In J. Knutson (Ed.), *Handbook of political psychology* (pp. 139–170). San Francisco: Jossey-Bass.

Sarbin, T. R. (1986). *Narrative psychology: The storied nature of human conduct.* New York: Praeger.

Schafer, R. (1992). *Retelling a life: Narration and dialogue in psychoanalysis.* New York: Basic Books.

Shipley, T., & Veroff, J. (1952). A projective measure of need for affiliation. *Journal of Experimental Psychology, 43,* 349–356.

Shneidman, E. S. (1992). Projections on a triptych or a hagiology for our time. In E. I. Megargee & C. D. Spielberger (Eds.), *Personality assessment in America: A retrospective on the occasion of the fiftieth anniversary of the Society for Personality Assessment* (pp. 87–95). Hillsdale, NJ: Erlbaum.

Smith, C. P. (Ed.). (1992). *Motivation in psychology: Handbook of thematic content analysis.* New York: Cambridge University Press.

Spence, D. P. (1982). *Narrative truth and historical truth: Meaning and interpretation in psychoanalysis.* New York: Norton.

Stein, M. I. (1981). *The Thematic Apperception Test: A manual for its clinical use with adults* (2nd ed., 2nd printing). Springfield, IL: Charles C Thomas. (Available from Mews Press, Box 2052, Amagansett, NY 11930)

Stewart, A. J. (1982). *Motivation and society.* San Francisco: Jossey-Bass.

Teglasi, H. (1993). *Clinical use of storytelling: Emphasizing the TAT with children and adolescents.* Boston: Allyn & Bacon.

Westen, D. (1991). Social cognition and object relations. *Psychological Bulletin, 109,* 429–455.

White, R. W. (1938). The case of Earnst. In H. A. Murray (Ed.), *Explorations in personality* (pp. 615–702). New York: Oxford University Press.

Winter, D. G. (1973). *The power motive.* New York: Free Press.

Winter, D. G., John, O. P., Stewart, A. J., Kohen, E. C., & Duncan, L. E. (1998). Traits and motives: Toward an integration of two traditions in personality research. *Psychological Review, 105,* 230–250.

Index

About the Editors

Lon Gieser, PhD, practices clinical psychology independently in Upper Montclair and Summit, NJ. He received his PhD from the Wright Institute at Berkeley, CA. Dr. Gieser's mentor was Nevitt Sanford, a colleague of Henry A. Murray, who helped develop the Thematic Apperception Test (TAT) at the Harvard Psychological Clinic. Dr. Gieser completed a post-doctoral internship at the University of Medicine and Dentistry of New Jersey, Newark, where he subsequently directed the Crisis Intervention Unit Short-Term Psychotherapy Clinic; later he directed adult outpatient psychological services at Fair Oaks Hospital in Summit, NJ. Dr. Gieser has been an editor for the *International Journal of Psychiatry in Medicine* and has published articles in other psychiatric journals. Dr. Gieser specializes in integrating personality assessment with treatment. His research interests include the history of psychology, authoritarianism, eating disorders, substance abuse, and academic underachievement. Dr. Gieser supervises psychotherapists, including graduate student interns from Seton Hall, Fairleigh Dickinson, and Montclair State Universities at COPE Counseling Center, Montclair, NJ, where he is a consulting psychologist. He is also a consultant to secondary schools and to Jespy House, Inc., a program for learning disabled adults in South Orange, NJ. In addition, Dr. Gieser is a community speaker and support group leader for the American Anorexia/Bulimia Association.

Morris I. Stein, PhD, is professor emeritus of psychology, New York University. Prior to that, he taught at the University of Chicago. He completed his undergraduate work at the College of the City of New York and earned his doctorate in social relations at Harvard University, where he was Murray's research assistant. During World War 2, Dr. Stein served in the assessment program of the Office of Strategic Services and has been a fellow at the Center for Advanced Study in the Behavioral Sciences. He also holds a Career Award from the National Institute of Mental Health. In 1996, he was awarded a Lifetime Career Award by the Creative Education Foundation for his research on creativity. In 1948, he published his first manual on the TAT, which was expanded and revised in 1955 to *The Thematic Apperception Test: An Introductory Manual for Its Clinical Use With Adults.* Following Murray's emphasis on the anabolic function of personality, Dr. Stein has been for many years involved in research on creativity—a topic on which he has lectured worldwide. His books on creativity include *Creativity and the Individual: Summaries of Selected Writings in the Psychological and Psychiatric Literature* (with S. J. Heinze; 1960); *Stimulating Creativity, Vol. I: Individual Procedures* (1974), and *Vol. II: Group Procedures* (1975); and *Gifted, Talented and Creative Young People: A Guide to Theory, Teaching and Research* (1984; all by Mews Press). In 1984, Dr. Stein also published *Making the Point: Anecdotes, Poems & Statements About the Creative Process* (Winslow Press), which to date has been translated into eight languages.

About the Cover

Henry Murray, Christiana Morgan, and other Harvard Psychological Clinic staff searched magazines for evocative illustrations and photographs. If an image successfully stimulated projection in experimental trials, it was sometimes redrawn by Morgan. Her drawings were amazingly close copies of the originals, with only minor changes to simplify the pictures or make them more ambiguous.

Redrawing had the effect of homogenizing the various artistic styles and avoided copyright concerns. Photographs of the original illustrations or Morgan's redrawings were glued onto cardboard stock to produce the early series of TAT cards.

"Picture C" was used in the first version of the Thematic Apperception Test (TAT) in the early 1930s but was not retained for use in later versions. Its history and origin were traced by one of this book's contributors, the indefatigable Wesley Morgan.

Picture C came from a 1931 *Woman's Home Companion* magazine illustration by Pruett Carter for Margaret Deland's "Captain Archer's Daughter," an abridged novel serialization. The illustration shows Mattie Archer and her husband Isadore Davis in a cabin aboard a tall-masted ship he owns. Some months earlier, Mattie had eloped with Isadore after a 4-day romance. She has just discovered that she is pregnant and wants to tell Isadore but finds him "in the dark nasty cabin which reeked with the smell of whiskey and pulsed with his slobbering snores." The illustration was captioned, " 'Why did I marry him?' She said dazed, 'Why?'"

A comparison of the original magazine illustration with Morgan's redrawing reveals that a porthole was changed into a window and that other details, such as 19th-century dress ornamentation and a flask and table by the bed, were eliminated. A vented passage door was redrawn as a four-panel wooden door to further obscure the picture's nautical origin.

The two-color illustration clipped from the magazine and Morgan's pen and ink drawing of the illustration were recovered from a wastebasket by Harvard Psychological Clinic staff member David Ricks during a 1956 clinic move. Ricks also found other original pictures and drawings for the TAT. Murray had no apparent interest in the materials and later rebuffed a gift of three of those pictures and drawings that Ricks had framed. Ricks later donated the framed works to the Henry A. Murray Research Center at Harvard University when it was established in 1976.